Praise for
How to Make Love to Adrian Colesberry:

"Like everyone else who picks up this book, I am now ready, yearning, and yes, demanding to go to bed with Adrian Colesberry. Bravo!" —Susie Bright

"If you've ever read *Our Bodies, Ourselves* and thought, 'But what about Adrian Colesberry's body? And what of Adrian Colesberry's self?' this hilarious guide is the book you've been waiting for." —Bob Powers, stand-up comic and author of *Happy Cruelty Day!*

"*How to Make Love to Adrian Colesberry* is one of the best books I have read on how to make love to Adrian Colesberry." —Marc Maron, stand-up comic and author of *The Jerusalem Syndrome*

"'Hats off to Adrian Colesberry,' I say (and bras and panties, too), for writing such a funny and delightful romp. And it makes me happy to know that I am now fully prepared to not only meet but thoroughly greet Adrian Colesberry, should I have the opportunity to come face-to-penis with him one day." —*Dish* magazine

"*How to Make Love to Adrian Colesberry* by Adrian Colesberry is a brilliant play on the Pale Fire slash Whatever for Dummies slash Disaster Handbook model, and a brilliant insight into modern love, to boot." —The Naughty Bride

"Never has a man written so evocatively and so lovingly about his penis. Of course, if all of us had penises like Adrian Colesberry's, I'm sure we'd want to write a guidebook as well. This is an indispensible book, even if you have no plans to make love to Adrian Colesberry. Serving suggestion: read aloud to your loved one in bed." —William McKeen, author of *Outlaw Journalist*

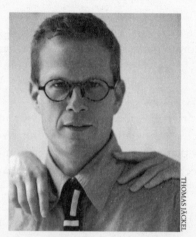

THOMAS JACKEL

Adrian Colesberry has a degree in biomedical engineering and spent ten years in pharmaceutical manufacturing. He now works as a movie extra and stand-up comic in Los Angeles, where he also does volunteer work teaching sex ed to high school students.

How to Make Love to® Adrian Colesberry

ADRIAN COLESBERRY

GOTHAM
BOOKS

GOTHAM BOOKS
Published by Penguin Group (USA) Inc.
375 Hudson Street, New York, New York 10014, U.S.A.

Penguin Group (Canada), 90 Eglinton Avenue East, Suite 700, Toronto, Ontario M4P 2Y3, Canada (a division of Pearson Penguin Canada Inc.); Penguin Books Ltd, 80 Strand, London WC2R 0RL, England; Penguin Ireland, 25 St Stephen's Green, Dublin 2, Ireland (a division of Penguin Books Ltd); Penguin Group (Australia), 250 Camberwell Road, Camberwell, Victoria 3124, Australia (a division of Pearson Australia Group Pty Ltd); Penguin Books India Pvt Ltd, 11 Community Centre, Panchsheel Park, New Delhi–110 017, India; Penguin Group (NZ), 67 Apollo Drive, Rosedale, North Shore 0632, New Zealand (a division of Pearson New Zealand Ltd); Penguin Books (South Africa) (Pty) Ltd, 24 Sturdee Avenue, Rosebank, Johannesburg 2196, South Africa
Penguin Books Ltd, Registered Offices: 80 Strand, London WC2R 0RL, England

Published by Gotham Books, a member of Penguin Group (USA) Inc.

Previously published as a Gotham Books hardcover edition

First trade paperback printing, July 2010

10 9 8 7 6 5 4 3 2 1

Gotham Books and the skyscraper logo are trademarks of Penguin Group (USA) Inc.

The Library of Congress has catalogued the hardcover edition of this book as follows:
Colesberry, Adrian
How to make love to Adrian Colesberry / by Adrian Colesberry.
    p. cm.
ISBN 978-1-592-40422-3 (hardcover) 978-1-592-40556-5 (paperback)
1. Sex—Humor. I. Title.
PN6231.S54C57 2009
818'.602—dc22   2008055556

How to Make Love to® is a registered trademark of Adrian Colesberry

Printed in the United States of America
Set in Minion • Designed by Sabrina Bowers

While the author has made every effort to provide accurate telephone numbers and Internet addresses at the time of publication, neither the publisher nor the author assumes any responsibility for errors, or for changes that occur after publication. Further, the publisher does not have any control over and does not assume any responsibility for author or third-party Web sites or their content.

WELCOME

Congratulations on your interest in how to make love to Adrian Colesberry! You will no doubt cherish your ability to make love to him for many years to come. You have your own personal reasons for wanting to learn how to make love to Adrian Colesberry. In case you forget later on, please take a moment to jot down a few notes here.

I, _____, want to learn how to make love to Adrian Colesberry because _____
_____
_____
_____
_____
_____
_____

Enjoy your Adrian Colesberry experience!

CONTENTS

A NOTE TO THE READER

Adrian's testicles are very sensitive.

If he could magically have you know one single thing about him before your clothes came off, that would be it. He's not freakishly hyperconcerned with the sensitivity of his testicles. Not at all. It's just that in the past, they've caused him some discomfort, which he'd like to avoid in the future if he could manage it.

"Easy enough," the plainspoken reader might be thinking. "Adrian should say, 'Before I take my pants off, I want you to know that my testicles are very sensitive.'"

Sounds simple. Maybe this fresh breath of honesty would inspire something like the following exchange:

You: Sensitive? Well, thanks for telling me.

Adrian: Sure thing.

You: So, kissing but no squeezing?

Adrian: Right.

You: While we're talking . . . my nipples are sensitive too.

Adrian: Let me guess . . . sucking and licking but no pinching?

You: Why, yes. You really understand me.

Adrian: And you understand me.

You: Now that we've had this refreshingly honest conversation, I'm hotter than ever for you.

Adrian: Likewise.

On the other hand, you might come back with, "Testicles? What made you think I was going to touch your testicles in the first place?!" Way too risky for Adrian Colesberry.

But what if you didn't have to learn about his testicles in the context of an awkward and potentially mood-wrecking conversation? What if there existed some reliable source, like a book, where you could read, as a matter of indifferent fact, that Adrian Colesberry's testicles were very sensitive? Then your knowledge of how to handle them properly would be just another skill set in your possession, like long division or changing a tire.

Luckily, such a reliable source does exist! It's *How to Make Love to Adrian Colesberry* (by Adrian Colesberry). And in addition to informing you that Adrian Colesberry's testicles are very sensitive, it's chock full of helpful examples of how to make love to Adrian Colesberry gathered from the real-life and mostly positive experiences of people—people just like you—making love to Adrian Colesberry.

A WORD ON VOCABULARY

Technically, there is no cursing in this book, not even the mildest curses like "heck" or "shoot." So if you find yourself offended by the excesses of popular music lyrics or the profanities used on television programs, relax. You'll find no such loose language here. At the same time, only the most robust words in the English language are used in reference to fun parts and sex acts. To make this distinction perfectly clear: The word "asshole" is never used to mean a disagreeable person, but is generously employed in reference to the body's back exit (or entrance, as you will).

There is one exception to this rule: Adrian Colesberry has forbidden the use of the language's strongest word for lady parts. Much like some ancient religions made it taboo to speak or write the name of their god, Adrian would not allow his most favored word for his most favored part of the human form to be used as a common reference in print.

Four words will be used in its place, because four words are required to match its strength: snatch, box, hole, and pussy (the last only in the context of oral intercourse).

THE QUICK-START GUIDE TO ADRIAN COLESBERRY

In case you can't wait to read a whole book before making love to Adrian Colesberry, this section provides some basic safety and handling tips. After using this guide to start out, be sure to read the detailed instructions that follow to ensure maximum enjoyment of Adrian Colesberry.

Testicles

Adrian Colesberry's testicles are very sensitive.

Arousal

Under normal operating conditions, Adrian Colesberry can be adequately aroused by tongue kissing. If you encounter Adrian Colesberry's shy penis, do not panic. Keep making out with him. If that doesn't work, just have him go down on you some more.

Make-Up Sex

Adrian Colesberry is unable to achieve an erection for at least twelve hours after a fight, a relationship talk, or any form of crying. Because of this feature, Adrian Colesberry is not equipped for make-up sex. There is no hardware or software upgrade that can be obtained to override this limitation.

Power Sources

Adrian Colesberry should be fed only the type of food indicated by Adrian Colesberry. If you are not sure what type of food is in your home, consult your roommate or your mother. If you intend to operate Adrian Colesberry for an extended time without food, refer to Adrian Colesberry.

Control

Use only those methods of control that are covered by these operating instructions. Aggressive, passive-aggressive, or other unauthorized methods may result in damage and will often require extensive work by a qualified technician or by Adrian Colesberry to restore Adrian Colesberry to his normal operation.

Modifications

Do not attempt to change any part of Adrian Colesberry. Your authority to operate Adrian Colesberry could be voided if you make changes or modifications not expressly approved by Adrian Colesberry.

LEGAL DISCLAIMERS

Adrian Colesberry makes no representations concerning any endeavor to review the content or any of the information (collectively, the "Materials") contained in or discussed in *How to Make Love to Adrian Colesberry*. You hereby acknowledge that any reliance upon the Materials shall be at your own risk. Adrian Colesberry does not make any warranty, express or implied, or assume any legal liability or responsibility for the accuracy, completeness, usefulness, legality, or decency of any information, apparatus, product, or process disclosed, or represent that its use would not infringe upon privately owned rights. Adrian Colesberry respects the rights of others. If you believe that your rights have been infringed upon in any way, please desist immediately from reading the Materials and/or interacting with Adrian Colesberry.

When used in the Materials, the words "love," "fuck," "cum," "erection," "orgasm," and similar expressions are intended to identify physical and/or emotional potentialities. Such concepts are subject to risks and uncertainties that could cause actual results to differ materially from those projected. Factors that could cause or contribute to the achievement of such potentialities include timely development of a sexual or emotional attachment that is sufficiently motivating to Adrian Colesberry, receipt of necessary verbal or nonverbal approvals, maintenance of sufficient psychological health and other factors set forth in various works of nonfiction and fiction, including but not limited to *Costa Rica: The Last Country the Gods Made*, *How to Make Love to Adrian Colesberry* (by Adrian Colesberry), several screenplays, a few speculation scripts for television situation comedies, and almost four hundred pages of an unfinished novel titled *The Perfect Freedom of Strangers*.

Adrian Colesberry undertakes no obligation to publicly release the result of any revision to these statements that may be made to reflect the occurrence of unanticipated events. The views and opinions of Adrian Colesberry do not necessarily state or reflect those of Adrian Colesberry.

How to Make Love to
Adrian Colesberry

Am I Right for Adrian Colesberry?

It breaks Adrian's heart when he thinks of the lost opportunities caused by people failing to mention that they'd like to make love to him.

Not that he's incapable of expressing his own desires. Far from it. Here's the problem: Adrian would like to have sex with practically everyone. Within five seconds of setting eyes on a woman, not only has the thought, "I'd fuck her!" run through his mind but in addition he's most likely sketched out several entertaining and mutually pleasurable sexual activities they could engage in together. You'll agree that it would occupy an unreasonable portion of his day to go around sharing these thoughts with every other person he ran into.

Some readers might be thinking, "Sounds nice, but Adrian wouldn't want to fuck me." Don't do that to yourself; Adrian's sexual interests are remarkably broad. Extensive research into his sexual history shows no patterns, proclivities, or standards. To illustrate this, Adrian's historical sexual partners are analyzed in six areas where some men can be quite picky in their sexual preferences: body style, ethnicity, experience, breast size, grooming, and hygiene.

Body Style

Here are hard numbers regarding the body styles of the eleven women Adrian Colesberry has slept with.

	WEIGHT (LBS)[1]	HEIGHT (FT)	BODY MASS INDEX
Adrian	165	5' 10"	23.7
Mean	127.8	5' 4 1/4"	21.8
Median	122.5	5' 4 1/2"	20.8
High	170.0	5' 7"	28.3
Low	98.0	4' 10"	18.8
Standard Deviation	19.97	2 1/2"	3.03

For those readers with a mathematical background, you can all too clearly perceive from this table Adrian's generous breadth of taste in body types. For those who require a more visual presentation, see the chart on page 3. If Adrian obeys statistical norms, 68.3 percent of his women will fall within the interior-most, "bull's-eye" section; 95.5 percent will fall within that and the surrounding unshaded section; and 99.7 percent will fall somewhere on the graph, just not in the black.

Each of Adrian's lovers and Adrian himself has been called out on the graph. (He's the bold-outlined square punching in at 5'10", 165 lbs.) Take a pen and draw yourself in. Even if your body doesn't land inside Adrian's "bull's-eye," don't fret. Look at those outliers: the 4'10", 100 lb. lady or the girl punching in at 5'7", 170. His libido has a significant weight and height range.

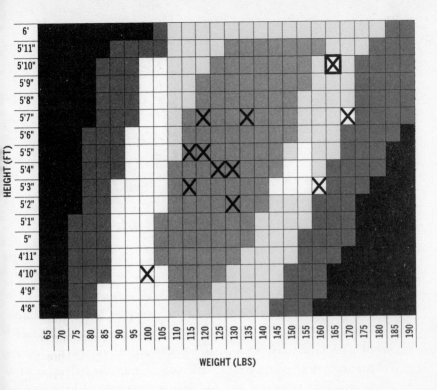

Ethnicity

Being himself a mixture of 62.5 percent German, 12.5 percent Italian, and 25 percent Southern White Trash, you might assume that Adrian would shy away from people of a less mongrel pedigree, but not at all. Five of the eleven women in his life have been of a sole lineage (one each of 100 percent Irish, Mexican, Jewish, Vietnamese, and Southern White Trash), with the remaining six of mixed origin. The chart on page 4 breaks down Adrian's historical ethnic experience.

ETHNIC ORIGIN

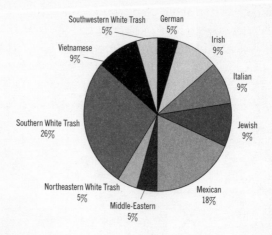

The chart seems to indicate a preference for Southern White Trash and Mexicans, but this is more properly seen as an artifact of his upbringing in a Southern border state.[2] Upon moving to an urban center on the West Coast, he folded in the Italian, Irish, Jewish, and Vietnamese in his new environment. Adrian fucks what he sees.

Experience

Adrian Colesberry has slept with eleven women in his life. If you have slept with fewer people, perhaps you worry that you're not experienced enough for him; if you have slept with more, perhaps you worry that he will think of you as some kind of whore.

Regarding inexperience, Adrian doesn't expect you to possess a mastery of sexual technique that could gain you profitable and enduring employment in a house of prostitution. Although if you do have some brothel-worthy skills, certainly do not omit them.

Keep in mind that Adrian isn't exactly one to be judgmental in this area. There are many women who would find him inexperienced. He will only ever expect of you what he demands of himself: enthusiasm and attention.

If you're worried about being too experienced, relax. While Adrian doesn't want to hear that you're fucking five other people at the time so will have to pencil him in on Thursdays between two and five, neither should it worry you if you somehow disclose the number of people you've been with in the past. He'll assume that you're the winner in this category unless you tell him otherwise.

And as for his thinking of you as some kind of whore, that's nothing but a good thing when properly applied, so keep it in your pocket for later.

Breast Size

Some men are particular in the area of breast size, but you needn't be concerned in this regard with Adrian Colesberry. He has experienced a wide range of breast sizes and enjoyed them all: A-cups account for 18 percent of his lovers, B-cups for 46 percent, and D-cups for 36 percent.

The C-cup-sized reader might note with alarm Adrian's lack of exposure to her specific breast size. True enough, he has no practical experience, but as seen already, all evidence points to him being adaptable. If he finds himself wandering about on the unfamiliar surface of a C-cup-sized breast, he will most likely survive by averaging the handling styles he has employed on D-cup- and B-cup-sized breasts.

The following graph of his lovers by bra cup illustrates his ability to engage with a wide range of breast sizes. [3]

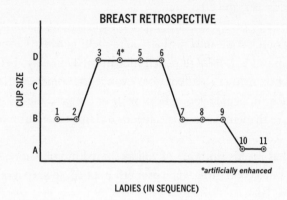

BREAST RETROSPECTIVE

CUP SIZE

*artificially enhanced

LADIES (IN SEQUENCE)

The mathematically oriented reader might be interested to observe that when you put a third-order polynomial best-fit line through this data set, it draws out the form of a woman's breast. If you're having trouble seeing it, turn the book 90 degrees counterclockwise. The line forms the unmistakable shape of a standing woman's breast in profile. Could this be a mere coincidence?[4]

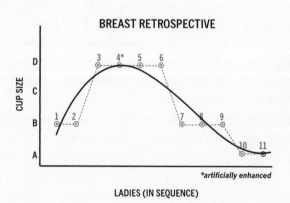

BREAST RETROSPECTIVE

CUP SIZE

*artificially enhanced

LADIES (IN SEQUENCE)

On first hearing the classic rhetorical question, "If somebody jumps off a cliff, would you jump after them?" neither the answer nor the intended life lesson was immediately apparent to Baby Adrian. From the questioner's tone of voice, he understood that he was supposed to enthusiastically respond in the negative, but in his heart, he had too many questions to embrace the expected answer.

How high is this so-called cliff? Is there a ledge that the jumper could cling on to? And what about the landing? Is it paved with pointy rocks, or is it a hillock of marshmallow pies that would cushion the longest fall like a sugary down pillow?

For obvious reasons, Adrian's parents endlessly worried that their son was too easily influenced by others. They were right, he was. But Adrian had a more positive slant on it. Instead of seeing himself as an alarmingly blank slate upon which anyone and everyone was invited to write, he saw himself as an adventurous joiner, as a radical democrat in his sources of inspiration.

Grooming

Traveling due south of the breast-size obstacle, the anxious reader might wonder, "Will Adrian like the way I shave (or don't shave) my lady parts?" Until recently, he held no preference one way or the other due to an insufficient sample size. But with his last six lovers Adrian has, purely by hazard, made love to an even sampling of the possible shaving styles: One-third of his recent lovers have been natural, one-third have only neatened their pubic hair without shaving, one-third have shaved themselves entirely clean and, the most important statistic, 100 percent of these six women have been able to make love to Adrian Colesberry.[5] Bottom line on grooming, then, is this: Shave your box or don't shave your box or neaten it up or leave it natural as you will. Adrian will adapt and he might even join you.

Smell

Adrian found out early in his career that he vastly preferred a woman's natural smell to that of any soap or perfume. In particular, he'll be interested in smelling your dirty hair.[6]

Recall that Napoleon asked Josephine to avoid the bath for two weeks before his return from campaign to court—so he could smell "her essence." That's all Adrian wants to do. Smell your essence. He's not a professional wine taster searching your scalp for overtones of maple syrup or nutmeg. He's not looking for any particular smell at all, just wants to learn your smell. You wouldn't wear a veil over your face when going out with Adrian Colesberry (unless you would, you kinky veil-faced lady), so don't hide your smell, either.

Genes

Adrian's father (by the gentleman's own admission) is "the biggest clean freak in the world." This might concern you about his son's abilities as a lover—sex being an activity where clean-freakishness puts you at a disadvantage. But the trait apparently doesn't pass in the genes. Unlike any anticipatable version of his father's son, Adrian enjoys in particular the earthy aspects of sex.

All the same, don't go as far as Josephine. Adrian doesn't want to fight through a cloud of funk or lick a crust of dirt off your body. He hasn't completely shaken off his culture's repulsion for natural odor; he just wants to take a half step back from it.

Tip: *If you want Adrian to love you, let him smell you. You. Not your favorite perfume or shampoo or shower gel or, worst of all, douche. You. You know the smell that soap ads say is bad? That smell.*

Your Ugliest Part

Despite all of these reassurances about Adrian Colesberry's breadth of taste in body style, breast size, ethnicity, grooming habits, and personal smell, you will still, most likely, enter the relationship shouldering one or two insecurities. Know this: Adrian will make it his hobby, nay, his obsession to take these off your back. If you're thinking, "Oh, how kind." Not at all. He does it more for himself than for you.

According to Adrian's logic, every insecurity you have about your body takes items off the menu of lovemaking. You think your ass is too big—lose the left half of the menu. Don't like your breasts, lose the back of the menu. You think you're not sexy, period—there's no menu at all; he just sits there sucking the mint flavor out of a toothpick. Adrian doesn't want any part of that. He wants you to be a full-on deli menu with breakfast served all day long.[7]

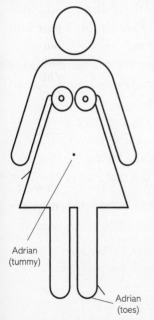

Adrian
(tummy)

Adrian
(toes)

The way he's worked things out—he will determine which part of your body you think is the least attractive, the most awkward, the part that embarrasses you, then he will target that part for special attention. This will communicate to your brain, "Adrian thinks my body is sexy, faults and all."

The confused reader may be thinking, "I thought that fucking me was enough to tell me that my body was sexy." No, fucking won't cut it. Straightforward sex says, "I like touching your boobs. I like fucking your snatch. I like it when you suck my cock." How not-at-all special.

Adrian can't imagine a snatch he wouldn't like to fuck. He'd enjoy touching most boobs, and everyone can suck his cock. If you count those activities as your only evidence that he wants to make love to you, you don't know whether he wants *you* at all. But when he makes love to your ugliest part, you will know for sure that it's *you* he wants to fuck. Take a moment to circle your ugliest part on the previous diagram. (You'll find already marked there the parts that Adrian thinks are his ugliest, in case you ever want to do anything about that.)

How Cute Do You Want to Be?

Maybe you're thinking, "It's nice and all that Adrian casts a wide net in his ability to love different types of women, but I want him to think that I personally am cute. Just me. Not a million other people too!" Here's where things get simple. Once you're fucking Adrian Colesberry the very thing that makes you cute to Adrian Colesberry is fucking Adrian Colesberry.

Apparently, some men work in the opposite way: They think a woman is desirable until they fuck her a few times, then not so much. It's like their cock is an eraser, fading the beauty they once saw. Adrian's cock works like a paintbrush that makes you more beautiful with every stroke.[8]

Tip: *If you want to get cuter to Adrian Colesberry, fuck him more. It's up to you. How cute do you want to be?*

Summary

Making love to Adrian Colesberry does not run through his penis. Adrian finds a girl who interests him and tells his penis to figure things out on the sex side. His penis has been performing this service reliably for years; relax in the knowledge that it will perform this service for you.

CHAPTER 1 NOTES

1   You might wonder how Adrian obtained accurate weight data for each of his girlfriends, seeing as women are not scrupulously honest when reporting this personal statistic, particularly to a lover. Four of these women did report their weight in contexts where the probability of lying seems unlikely, as in, "I gained 5 pounds over the holidays. Usually, I only weigh 125." As for the rest, Adrian has picked up or carried each of these women at one time or another. Granted, he is not and has never been a guess-your-weight operator at a carnival, but by comparing the perceived lightness of a woman of unknown weight to the perceived lightness of a previous woman of known weight, Adrian has been able to provide estimates of credible accuracy. (It must be mentioned that in the context of lovemaking, all women, and you will be no exception, feel light as air to Adrian Colesberry.)

2   Surprising that Adrian has failed to make love to any African American women, especially considering the fact that he was exposed to many black women in the Southern city of his youth, but it can be easily explained: Upon learning of the centuries-long tradition of white men sexually exploiting black women, Teen Adrian resolved to never impose his sexuality in any form on the black women of his own generation. In his late twenties, he got over this block. He knew that he'd gotten over it because upon seeing a black woman, he'd think, "Oh, I'd fuck her!" and then he'd sketch out several entertaining and mutually pleasurable sexual activities they could engage in together.

Once he started getting these feelings, he couldn't act on them because he was married, but, for the record, he did go out with an African American woman after his divorce. While they never made love in the full meaning of the term, he did spend a delightful morning massaging her snatch.

3

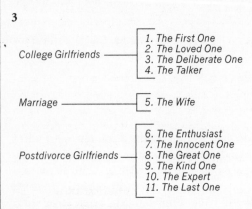

College Girlfriends
1. The First One
2. The Loved One
3. The Deliberate One
4. The Talker

Marriage
5. The Wife

Postdivorce Girlfriends
6. The Enthusiast
7. The Innocent One
8. The Great One
9. The Kind One
10. The Expert
11. The Last One

4   The answer is yes; it not only could be but definitely is a coincidence. Yet, it does make the shape of a breast, which is lovely.

5   Adrian had his first chance to develop an opinion on the topic of shaving while on his third date with the Enthusiast, his first girlfriend after his divorce. From the way she draped herself over her furniture and his body, Adrian thought he was going to get lucky after their first date. He was wrong. She held them strictly to making out—like they were being chaperoned by a nun. Wouldn't even let him unbutton her shirt. Then at the end of their third date, she and Adrian ended up drunk on her couch and after only a few minutes of making out, she allowed them to go beyond kissing and outside-the-shirt boob handling. Adrian unbuttoned her top. She helped him take off her bra. He massaged her boobs for long enough not to appear overeager, then he unzipped her khakis and pushed his intoxicated fingers below her waistband. This was going to be the first strange snatch he'd felt in fifteen years.

He got halfway to her knee before realizing he'd overshot.

To give her the impression that his incompetent groping was part of a sensual master plan, Adrian gripped her thigh and jiggled it as if to say, "Now that's a thigh!"

Tip: *Take the lead from Adrian here. Regardless of what you do in bed, act like it's exactly what you meant to do. You didn't submit a flight plan after all. Keep that poker face, and Adrian will think you meant to lick his eye—you crazy, kinky eye-licker.*

Once he'd gotten his bearings, Adrian headed back up the inside of her leg, paying careful attention this time. As soon as his fingers tripped over her labia, he realized why he'd missed it on his first pass—the Enthusiast had shaved herself completely clean.

"What happened to pubic hair?" he wondered. It's not like Adrian was totally out of the know on hairlessness. He'd seen bald women in pornos and realized that women had to shave or wax to wear those tiny bathing suits. It just surprised him that a civilian would shave hers bare for a normal date with a normal guy like him, Adrian Colesberry.

Overcoming his initial surprise, he quickly got used to the new feel and enjoyed himself so thoroughly that, by the time he left the next morning, bald snatches were A-OK by him.

But more interesting than his reaction or nonreaction to the Enthusiast's presentation of her pubic hair is what he did next: Adrian drove home and shaved his balls. Why, you ask? Because Adrian Colesberry is a joiner. (See sidebar, page 7.)

That next Saturday, the Enthusiast did him the favor of licking his newly depilated testicles. Adrian didn't really like it better than he had before and, for her part, the Enthusiast wasn't wowed by the change in terrain, at least not enough to mention it. You'd think that their mutual indifference to his shaving would have prompted Adrian to abandon the project, but no. He continued to shave for the remaining weeks of their relationship.

Whichever of your habits Adrian has latched onto—genital shaving, wearing too much cologne, drinking to excess, not eating carbs, only eating carbs—it will be equally unimportant whether he likes to do them or whether you even want him to do these things with you. He'll just enjoy the fact that you're on the same team—a team that stinks a lot or drinks a lot or eats carbs or not, or one that hits the shower and scrapes hair off their fun bits before getting together to fuck. That's Adrian's kind of team.

6   Adrian discovered his love for a woman's natural smell from the Loved One, his second girlfriend from his college years. A few days after their first date, she called to ask him if she could come over the next Friday and have Adrian wash her hair. Adrian is nothing if not a good sport, so he said, "Sure! No problem." One week later, he sat her in a straight-backed walnut chair, tipped it against his sink and gently arranged her hair in the bowl. Up to the moment when he turned the tap on, he'd thought of her request as a childish game in which he was kindly indulging her. When the first handful of warm water hit her scalp, he understood.

The smell of her dirty hair filled his tiny bathroom; nearly smothering him. In one breath, he felt closer to the Loved One than he'd ever felt to anyone outside his own family, and he hadn't even kissed her yet. After that night, he would get horny at just a whiff of her scalp. The Loved One sure knew what she was up to.

Tip: Dirty reader, definitely ask Adrian to lather-rinse-repeat your hair. He's down for it and it ends up being a brilliant move, as you've seen.

Adrian had forgotten the lesson of the dirty hair when, eighteen years later, he found himself unable to engage like he wanted to with the Great One (his epochal third girlfriend after the divorce). But even though his brain didn't remember, his nose did: Every time they met, he'd bury his face in the Great One's hair and take in a lungful. Only the obliging woman would invariably have washed it the night before in anticipation of their date, so it only ever smelled like tea-tree oil or tropical fruit salad. You can imagine his frustration.

Once he realized what he was after, he asked the Great One to avoid washing her hair so close to their get-togethers. She was kind enough to back off her shampoo day to earlier in the week and the next time they hooked up, it was like meeting her for the first time.

7   Adrian developed his Ugliest Part theory several years into his marriage. The Wife had put on a few pounds, so he got the idea that her weight was the thing slowing down their sex life. In reality, it had crawled to a stop years before, but in his optimistic delusion he imagined that her negative body image was the only problem they had. He started being physically affectionate to her tummy and helped her buy new clothing so she would feel better about herself. That did make the Wife feel more accepted, but acceptance was all she wanted, so it didn't get Adrian laid more.

After the divorce, Adrian dusted off his theory when he noticed that the Enthusiast was self-conscious about her ass—to the point that she never let him look at it. To go to the bathroom, she'd wrap herself in a sheet and back away from the bed, like in old movies. He blew it off as a manageable quirk until he realized that they'd never fucked doggie-style. Clearly, this had to end.

Ass-conscious reader, there are two main things Adrian likes to look at while he's fucking you: your face and your ass. He doesn't have elaborate preconceptions about what your ass should look like. He just likes to look at the ass that he's fucking while he's fucking it. He's deeply sorry that it's no longer the ass you had in high school. He wishes he'd have been around back then to see that ass, but he still wants to see the ass that you have now.

One night, right after she'd returned from her backward walk to the bathroom, Adrian flipped the Enthusiast onto her stomach and fucked her from behind while fondling her buttocks. A woman who doesn't want you to see her ass from across a room really doesn't like you eyeballing it point-blank. It worked, though. After a few goes in that position, it got through to the Enthusiast that Adrian couldn't be that disgusted by her big ass if he still had an erection to push inside her.

His Ugliest Part theory met with equal success when he applied it to his next girlfriend, the Innocent One, and her body hair issues, but he ran into a problem when he got to the Great One: She had no obvious physical insecurities, so she became the first person to be asked the Ugliest Part question outright.

Instead of giving him a proper answer to his perfectly reasonable inquiry, the Great One responded, "Why would you ask such a stupid question?"

Lying, Adrian said he didn't know.

Way too clever for that evasion, the Great One guessed that for him to ask the question, he must have a part of his own body that he didn't like. He hadn't seen it that way, but . . . yes! Her logic was flawless. It would certainly explain why he'd gotten so obsessed with his Ugliest Part strategy—he had staged the whole thing to encourage someone to ask him about his own ugliest part.

It's his toes and a little bit his tummy, even though he doesn't have much of one. Adrian picked up the ridiculous thing about his toes from the Wife. They're not unattractive, just long, but she somehow made him think they were ugly by constantly saying, "You have the ugliest toes!" She wasn't being mean as much as she was soliciting compliments for her own toes, which were shorter than his.

The Great One listened patiently to his deeply touching, low toe-esteem story, but she never made love to his feet, so Adrian put his Ugliest Part theory back on the shelf. Then a week later, he had just finished going down on her when she mentioned, in as casual a voice as she could find, "I think I have long labia for a girl. Do you think so?"

In unnecessarily qualifying her question with, "for a girl" the Great One wasn't reminding Adrian that only girls had labia; she was petitioning him, in the sweetest possible way, to keep in mind while formulating his answer that she was herself a girl. Adrian heard her loud and clear.

Before making a judgment on how she compared to the general population in the category of labial length, or at least that population as experienced by Adrian Colesberry, he went down on her again. If someone asks for his opinion on the wine, he takes another sip before commenting.

Since she had brought it up, yeah, he supposed that her labia were longer than some. He didn't say so, of course, and never would have—to a girl. What he did was draw up his head and report that the Wife's had been longer, which was true, so he wouldn't likely have noticed the relative lengthiness of her own. This, combined with his spirited-as-always cunnilingus, seemed to make her feel more secure about her labia. At least she didn't have any more questions on the topic.

Then it dropped on him like an anvil: Right when he'd given up on finding out what the Great One's ugliest part was, she'd up and blurted it out. And it was her snatch!

Dear reader, if you think the ugliest part of your body is your box, you've got it made with Adrian Colesberry. And while you're squatting over a mirror trying to work out your aesthetic criticisms of that area, check to see if your asshole is as pretty as you think it should be. Not up to par, you say? Good deal. Adrian will be lifting your self-esteem in no time.

8   The Last One didn't understand the principle of making herself cute to Adrian by fucking him more when, a couple of months into their relationship, they hit a little dry spell. One evening, she emerged from the bathroom fully made up, wearing a fancy dress and heels. Adrian, who is capable of being a total idiot in these situations, asked her what the occasion was, and the Last One explained that she was just trying to look more feminine, on account of their dry spell.

She was right that her cute had worn off a bit, only her solution was flawed. If she wanted to rekindle her femininity in Adrian's mind, she could have saved herself all that preening and just sat on his face. (There's no vantage from which a woman appears more feminine to Adrian Colesberry than the view from between her legs.) Or if that felt too risky in the moment, she could have taken his cock out of his pants. That makes a woman especially pretty to Adrian.

CHAPTER 2.

Seducing Adrian Colesberry

Not to dampen your newly formed confidence about being a suitable candidate for Adrian Colesberry, but you're still not making love to him. (Unless you are making love to him already, in which case, congratulations. You can skip over this chapter.) Before you make love to him, you're going to have to meet him. To help you strategize, find below all available information about the various places he has met his previous lovers:

First the raw data (for researchers wishing to perform their own statistical manipulations).

LOVER	MEETING PLACE	PREROMANTIC RELATIONSHIP	TIME TO INTERCOURSE (DAYS)	RELATIONSHIP LENGTH (AFTER FIRST INTERCOURSE, DAYS)
1	Party/Bar	No	0	140
2	Party/Bar	No	25	845
3	Workplace	Yes	180	400
4	Friend of a friend's	Yes	45	90
5	Educational setting	Yes	21	5,475
6	Workplace	Yes	1,278	45
7	Creative setting	Yes	50	85
8	Educational setting	No	180	125
9	Creative setting	Yes	90	469
10	Party/Bar	No	6	75
11	Internet	No	24	1,606

Crunching the numbers reveals the frequency for each meeting place, the average days to intercourse, and the average relationship length after first intercourse, for each location and overall.

LOCATION	FREQUENCY %	TIME TO FIRST INTERCOURSE (DAYS)	RELATIONSHIP LENGTH (AFTER FIRST INTERCOURSE, DAYS)
Friend of a friend's	9	45	90
Internet	9	24	1,606
Creative setting	18	70	277
Educational setting	18	101	2,800
Workplace	18	729	223
Party/Bar	27	10	353

	DAYS TO FIRST INTERCOURSE	RELATIONSHIP LENGTH (AFTER FIRST INTERCOURSE, DAYS)
Average	173[1]	850
Median	45	140

In an attempt to cater to diverse learning styles, the data has been graphed.

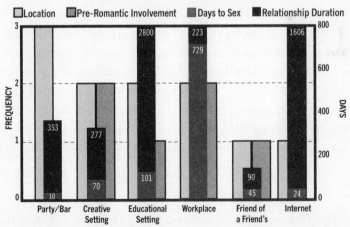

MEETING PLACE FREQUENCIES

For those who enjoy reading more than graph gazing, the following analysis is provided:

Preromantic or No? It turns out that you get neither an advantage nor a disadvantage by knowing Adrian before the romantic relationship starts. Fifty-five percent of his lovers did develop a preromantic relationship with Adrian. Forty-five percent went right to the romance.

The reader who likes to get to know someone before diving into the romantic portion of the relationship is advised to approach Adrian at the workplace, a creative setting, or a friend of a friend's. Those who want to dive right into the chase and pursuit should catch him at a party or bar or in a creative setting. The educational setting caters to either approach.

Straight to the Sex? Anyone who wants to get in Adrian's pants right away is advised to meet him at a party or bar.[2] It provides the minimal time to sexual contact and not a bad relationship length afterward. The workplace punches in as the obvious worst of all worlds: Not only do you have to wait forever to get a taste, but the relationship doesn't last so long afterward. (It's possible that Adrian develops an incestlike taboo regarding sexual contact with coworkers.)

The Long Game? If you're going for relationship length, clearly the educational setting and the Internet are the best candidates. As a student, Adrian is open to new inputs, and you're a new input. The Internet provides the most efficient way to start and maintain a long-term relationship with Adrian Colesberry. This should surprise precisely no one, since the Internet provides the most efficient way to do everything.

Getting Picked up by Adrian Colesberry

Adrian Colesberry is not a competent pickup artist. When the pressure's off, he can be confident and charming, but when the pressure is on, he cannot focus those attributes into a package that compels girls to come back to his place and fuck him. This doesn't apply to you, of course. You'll only have to listen to a minute of his self-effacing mumblings before you decide to step out of your panties for him. But that's you and your tigerlike perception. Most girls take a lot longer than that.

Turning lemons into lemonade, his incompetence plays to your advantage. A woman who hasn't read this book might not even know when Adrian is hitting on her, whereas you'll pick up on his subtle signals right away. At least you'll be familiar with his classic maneuver, the one where he palms you a business card and then runs off.[3]

A Note on the Party/Bar. Aware of his deficiencies in the area of picking up women, Adrian has sought out advice from pickup artists. Here's what he was taught:

1. Go to a bar or club early in the evening.
2. Grab a stool in the center of the bar.
3. Hit on all the girls who have to reach around you to get a drink.
4. Fuck anyone who will have you.

The plan is simple and primal, like a wild dog hanging out at a watering hole and jumping the bitches in heat when they finally get too thirsty to stay away. It worked well for the pickup master who taught it to him. Using this technique, the gentleman would draw drink-seeking girls into intense conversation and, most of the time, get laid for his trouble.

But if you want access to Adrian Colesberry in this environment, don't look for the quick-talking seduction of a pickup artist. His brand of dry humor is wasted in yell-talk—how clever can anything be on the third repeat and at the top of the lungs? Hold off for a bit until he gets drunk and starts looking for someone to dance with.[4] Then either ask him to dance yourself or, if that's not your bag, here's how to ensure that he'll ask you:

1. Determine the trajectory of his drunken search for a dancing partner.
2. Post up somewhere along his path.
3. Move to the music. Not full-on dancing as in, "I'm perfectly happy dancing with myself," but more like, "I can't help but move to this music and would welcome an invitation to continue moving opposite someone else."
4. He'll ask you to dance on his first pass.

It couldn't matter less how well you dance. It's hardly Adrian's best event. And if you're thinking that you'll embarrass yourself, don't worry, you will. That's exactly the point. Dancing and fucking are alike that way—if you're not doing anything that feels embarrassing, you're not trying hard enough.

What Adrian Colesberry Will Say About Himself

You have been so immersed in facts and strategies all revolving around Adrian Colesberry and how to make love to him that you quite understandably may have the misimpression that the real-life Adrian Colesberry thinks the entire world revolves around him, and that your first date with the man will be like living a chapter of this book in the flesh—amusing conversation about his habits and needs, peppered with some not-so-subtle hints about the sensitivity of his testicles, followed by some delightful lovemaking. Nothing could be further from the truth (except for the delightful lovemaking).

Checking Out Adrian Colesberry

Far from causing Adrian any anxiety, it will actually relieve him if you commit your tenth or third or even your first date together having him scrutinized by your aunt or older brother or that girlfriend who totally pegged your last boyfriend as a psycho-narcissist and you told her she was crazy but she was right: He was totally a psycho-narcissist and there's no way you're letting anyone, even Adrian Colesberry, into your pants without her approval.

Bring her along and anybody else who wants to come with her.[5] In his formative years, Baby Adrian attended a school where his mother was the headmistress. He spent every day of his childhood being scrutinized. As a result, being scrutinized is Adrian's best event.

The better move is not to bring anyone to check out Adrian on your first few dates. It's not that anything bad can come of it. It's just pointless. Bringing a friend or relative on a first date with Adrian Colesberry to make sure he passes muster is like bringing your pet cat on a first date with Saint Francis of Assisi to make sure he's good with animals.

The reason Adrian has cooperated in the writing of this book is precisely because he won't have the stomach to say much if anything about himself on your first date.[6] You know so much about him now that, aside from clearing up an item of confusion here and elaborating on a point of personal history there, you can spend your first happy hours together focused on you.[7]

What You Should Say About Yourself: The Real You

When he meets you, Adrian won't ask where you're from or what you do or where you go to school or any of the things people generally talk about when they meet. He's not interested in Frankensteining together a version of the real you from available evidence, like a detective profiling a serial killer. He's interested in experiencing a new person . . . new to him and maybe new to you, too.[8]

The way he sees it, either you can choose to spend your first minutes together trotting out the ready-to-wear version of who you are—the one you've been pulling on for years—or you can choose to tailor a new you right on the spot.

Bad Boyfriends Welcomed

Just like raw oysters are best served with a dash of hot sauce, Adrian Colesberry goes down better after at least one bad boyfriend. High school girls wanted nothing to do with him, preferring boys who looked and acted like they were going to take the world by storm. It's only after learning that those kinds of boys also take women by storm that women start looking at Adrian Colesberry through more sympathetic eyes. If you haven't yet had a bad boyfriend, that's OK too. Maybe you're smarter than most. By no means should you go out and get one just to enhance your enjoyment of Adrian Colesberry.

He's not encouraging you to make up some big story, like, "I'm the expatriated child of an Argentine general and I put myself through college by cashing in $150,000 worth of torture-extorted bearer bonds." But, say you're a gastroenterologist, and you start to tell him about what you do, and, right as the word "gastroenterologist" is forming on your lips, it suddenly pops into your brain how you collected butterflies in fourth grade until the other kids made such fun of you that you stopped. Just consider the possibility of skipping over your profession and telling him, "I like collecting butterflies." You could go to the museum of natural history on your first date and wander through the entomology exhibit.

Rightly or wrongly, Adrian will assume that you're taking advantage of this *new you* opportunity when you meet. Out of respect for your reinvention process, he won't put much stock in things you tell him about your past or about what you do when you're out there, away from him. He'll like hearing stories with you in them, but in the end, that's all they are—stories. The only knowledge of you that he'll trust will come from how you act around him.

Complimenting Adrian

Adrian is not the mangy dog at the pound or the whore with the heart of gold. He is a pleasant, well-mannered, considerate gentleman who makes great efforts to be an attentive listener and a witty conversationalist. It might dawn on you to make some kindly remarks on this topic, but don't. Most people do take a liking to him, so it will never surprise Adrian to learn that you do as well.

The pro tip is not to compliment him but to say that you're attracted to him for something he didn't work for at all, for something he just is and couldn't help being.[9] Tell Adrian you can't keep your hands off a guy who wears glasses. Tell him you're a sucker for hazel eyes. It's the difference between earning a hundred dollars and finding a hundred-dollar bill on the ground. Adrian likes it easy.

Best thing is that you don't have to break the ice with this whole strategy. Adrian will go first. Maybe he'll tell you that you have his favorite texture of hair or that you're the exact right height or that your breasts are the perfect size.

How does that make you feel? Maybe like you can stop trying so hard and relax? How could you not relax? By a natural accident, you have the perfect-sized breasts! Where's he going to find another pair exactly like those? Nowhere. That's where.

Touting Your Sexual Skills

By now, you may have calculated that the best approach for you personally is to convince Adrian right off the bat that you have something to offer him sexually. Directly marketing your sexual abilities is a decent choice. He'll enjoy hearing you talk dirty to him, but he won't put any stock in your promises. Just like you can't tell who's going to win a volleyball game by listening to the smack-talk beforehand, Adrian doesn't believe that pre-sex dirty talk reliably predicts behavior between the sheets.[10]

As far as he's concerned, it's a neutral signal, along with tramp stamps, tongue piercings, supershort skirts, or any other effort to market your sexual availability and enthusiasm—all that stuff is fun to listen to/look at, but they don't mean you'll deliver.

You could be marketing because you've got a truly great product, like a delicious organic coffee, and want people to know about it or you could be marketing because you've got something utterly worthless, like a sugared cola, and have to go to extraordinary efforts to make people buy it.

Public Behavior

When you and Adrian first start going out as a couple, you might notice that he acts a bit twitchy in public as compared to when you're in private. "Where," you might wonder, "is the calm self-mastery I've come to expect from this charming example of a man?" Rightly, you might entertain concerns that Adrian Colesberry has a social disorder or some tiresome phobia. Happily, he has neither.

He's not wrestling with any of his own demons. He's worrying about you: wondering whether you're a bizarre exhibitionist, a kleptomaniac, or maybe a complete nutcase.[11] When after a few dates, you've failed to turn into any of these things, he'll calm down. The partial exception to his public shyness is making out. Adrian can be maneuvered into making out with you in public, but you'd be advised to get him drunk first.[12]

Timing the Move

Adrian uses entirely conventional standards to decide when to kiss you, when to cop a feel, and when to sneak his hand down your pants. Review the following table to familiarize yourself with his state of mind and what activity he will initiate on which date. (Up until you fuck for the first time, he uses date-timing—not calendar-timing—to measure relationship time.)

Date	Internal Dialogue	Physical Activities He'll Initiate
1	*Ungentlemanly to try something now. Maybe she's just being polite. Might not even like me. If I try something, she'll think that I think she's a whore. That's bad. Don't do anything.*	*A relatively chaste kiss*
2	*Oh, she's back. Nice. I'll test the waters.*	*Mouth-to-mouth kissing, but not full-on making out. Touching face with back of fingers. Touching hand.*
3	*Back again?! Ungentlemanly not to try something now. If I don't try something, she'll think I don't want to fuck her. But I do want to fuck her. Do something!*	*Open-mouth kissing. Touching breasts with back of fingers, then front. Putting hand down pants. Oral sex. Fucking.*

You may have been puzzled by the maneuver where he touches your face and breasts with the back of his fingers. In Adrian's mind, the backs of the fingers are friendlier than the fronts when first touching a woman. It's still touching but it's not the part of his fingers that can go on to grab or unbutton or do anything that you might see as unwelcomed. If you're harboring any anxiety in the neighborhood of "What is he up to?" the back of his fingers communicate that it's just about the touch.[13]

Needless to say, you can easily modify this schedule such that things come later. Although Adrian is mentally capable of initiating sex on the third date, he won't turn into a robot, relentlessly pursuing sex just because it appears in the calendar in his brain. A word or a simple lack of enthusiasm will send Adrian to his end of the couch or to the door without a single protest.

Modifying the schedule in the other direction is not so easy. Adrian is impossibly poor at reading any subtle signals sent to encourage him in this direction. A slyly averted gaze, an insistent stare, a flirtatious giggle, even a hand placed on his forearm . . . all the signs that are used to invite a man to make his move are lost on him. So if you want him to cop a feel before your third date, good luck. You'll need it.[14]

Imaginative Foreplay

Adrian needs a little foreplay before foreplay. The foreplay he needs is called fucking. The sensitive reader might be shocked and disappointed by this genitally centered, unsensual, immature, cut-to-the-chase attitude toward sexuality. But before you go any further down that road, know that Adrian will engage in any foreplay you like, just fuck his brains out first.

You probably feel silly now for jumping to conclusions. Adrian Colesberry isn't any of those things you called him. Don't feel bad, though. Adrian would have said the same things once upon a time because, once upon a time, he was entertained by any and every sensual activity—a foot rub, a long bath, an especially lively conversation. Unfortunately, this model of Adrian Colesberry is no longer available.[15]

All is not lost, though; the current model will begin to relax about the whole thing once you've fucked him enough. He'll happily rub your feet or let you massage his back and when he starts finger-fucking you or handling your boobs, it'll be because he wants to, not because some egg timer in his head is going off to remind him that he should really be fucking you.

If, despite this happy ending, you still view his attitude as an impasse, here's a possible compromise between the different kinds of foreplay that you and Adrian require. If you have to cuddle, try cupping Adrian's balls while he cuddles you. Or if you have to talk, why don't you chatter away while sitting on his face? Just be sure to keep your legs generously spread so that your thighs don't block his ear holes. That way, he can listen to your each and every thesis and respond intelligently once you let him up for air.

He Can Only Make Love to What He Can See

Shy reader, the title of this section may make Adrian Colesberry seem unsympathetic to your need for darkness. No such thing. He completely understands why you want to make love in the dark. Maybe the dark helps you relax, or you feel self-conscious in full illumination, so you like to turn the lights off. Perfectly natural. No one wants to fuck under interrogation lamps.[16]

Adrian isn't saying that your preference for the dark is wrong, he's just asking you to abandon it as long as you're fucking him. For Adrian Colesberry, fucking in the dark is like eating in the dark. He can do it. He just doesn't know why he'd want to. As long as he can remember, he's liked to see what he's fucking, probably because he learned about sex from pornography.[17]

The insecure reader might be intimidated by the idea of Adrian's mentally comparing her body to some twenty-year-old porn girl's. Rest easy. Porn girls separate themselves from the pack less by their beauty or well-toned bodies than by their well-lit exhibitionism. If you're willing to allow Adrian a leisurely look between your legs in adequate light, you've immediately brought yourself up to par.

"But what if he doesn't like the way mine looks?"

Perish the thought.

Thanks to pornographers' documentarian-like interest in variety and detail, Adrian has seen hundreds of different snatches—up close and larger than life—wet and dry, large and small, bald and bushy, propped invitingly open and demurely closed. He has enjoyed looking at every snatch that has passed in front of his eyes; he'll certainly enjoy looking at yours.

CHAPTER 2 NOTES

1   Adrian's long preromantic acquaintanceship with the Enthusiast (see row 6 in the table on page 18) raises the average time to intercourse up to 173 days, nearly a half a year. He was married when they met, so nothing was consummated until after the marriage ended. When forming your own expectations about how long it will take you to break yourself off a chunk of Adrian Colesberry, observe the median time to intercourse of forty-five days.

2   If you're imagining that alcohol accounts for Adrian being such fast work in a bar, this is not the case. He was dead sober in two of his three bar/party hookups.

3   Right after he got divorced, Adrian went to a lot of pottery workshops. After a couple of months with no results, he gave up on it as a way to get laid, which is funny, looking back, since he'd snagged the brass ring on his first time around without even knowing.

At the very first class he attended, he ran into two girls. They flirted for a while afterward until the place started thinning out. Then that moment came when he could have suggested that they all go for coffee, and they'd have been like, "Yeah, let's go." That didn't happen, but he did palm each girl a business card then ran away like a third-grader who'd been kissed.[*]

Half a year after that first workshop, one of the girls e-mailed Adrian out of the blue, wondering if he wanted to go out. It took him a while to recall their meeting, and once he did he couldn't remember which one she was.

He started to compose an e-mail asking her to send him a photo, but then he thought, "Wait a second! Who cares what precisely she looks like?" The way he figured it, six months ago, she'd

---

[*] *In Adrian's head the card-and-run strategy was respectful to the liberated modern woman who had the right to give her number or not. It did indeed liberate them from ever having anything else to do with Adrian Colesberry.*

been cute enough for him to flirt with. Unless she'd been busy that whole time making herself ugly . . .

He wrote her back saying how delighted he was that she had *finally* contacted him and how he'd be thrilled to go out with her. If she hadn't had the perception to recognize that Adrian was hitting on her super-hard when he handed her that business card then ran off, he would have missed the relationship that completely changed his life. This was the Great One.

4 The Wife hated dancing, and the few times he got her to go with him, he didn't much like dancing either because she only ever wanted to do what she called the Bump. He'd never learned to do the Bump, but that was OK because she taught him. It's pretty easy. You stand side-by-side and slam your hips together with increasing force—like a demolition derby with your ass. Miserable.

One year, they took dancing lessons in the hope of reinjecting some romance into the marriage. They quickly fell far behind the rest of the class, which was hard to do since most of them were hopelessly uncoordinated misfits who had never danced in their lives and were only there so that they could competently execute the first dance at their own wedding reception after which they would never dance again, including any further dancing at their own wedding reception.

Around week four, the instructor helpfully pointed out why Adrian and the Wife had become the flunkies in a class of flunkies—the Wife wasn't following Adrian's lead. If he led her to the right, she'd move to the left.

"Wait," the freedom-loving reader might object, "by what law does she have to follow him?" Technically, of course, she has to follow him by the laws of ballroom dancing, but the Wife couldn't bring herself to do anything Adrian asked her to do, even if it was only for one hour a week and in the context of a dancing class that she herself had signed them up for.

In an effort to salvage the Wife's strategy for salvaging their marriage, Adrian suggested that she take the lead. Only, she couldn't lead any better than she could follow. If she moved to the right, the very fact that he followed made her change her mind and move to the left. Their marital problems didn't have a lot of subtext to them.

5 His first date with the Great One was a dinner with her aunt. The Last One took him to meet friends on the fourth date and had him crossing the continent to meet her brother and his family within a month. Needless to say, he passed all these tests with flying colors.

If you really want to check out Adrian Colesberry, instead of putting him into good-behavior mode, put him on his worst behavior: Drain his rather deep well of cheery goodwill and observe the man he will be in the rough patches that will inevitably crop up if you hang around for long enough. But how, you wonder, can you do this without yourself looking like an agitator? Answer: Take him to an amusement park. While you enjoy the high-velocity rides and non-nutritious food, Adrian will be reliving one of the worst moments of an all-but-constantly miserable marriage. The details are unimportant, but . . . the Wife, ignoring repeated requests by the swing-carousel ride operator to stop grabbing at Adrian's legs, made the ride stop, got them both ejected, and in his first and only full-scale panic attack, Adrian finally decided to get a divorce. If you can like Adrian Colesberry at an amusement park, just face it: You like Adrian Colesberry.

6 Adrian hasn't always been prudent enough to stay mum about the Wife. He talked the poor Enthusiast's ear off. Their mutually agreed-upon breakup, though definitely catalyzed by other failures, was mainly caused by his inability to shut up about his ex-wife. He didn't make that mistake again. Neither the Innocent One nor the Great One ever heard a peep, and you won't either, at least not at first.

You have to admit that if you were five years in and he'd never talked about her, that'd be creepy, like he'd killed her. He didn't do anything like that. So needless to say, if you hang around for long enough, you'll hear not just about the Wife but about every other lousy thing that ever happened to him. In return, he will, of course, be happy to listen to every lousy thing that ever happened to you.

7 For the sake of clarity, in this sentence, while the second-to-last you meant you two, the all-important final you meant you singular, or the person on the date who is not Adrian Colesberry. When you go on that epic first date, the you that you call me is the one you two will be focused on.

8   The Loved One from back in college took full advantage of Adrian's New You policy. He knew next to nothing about her, and she chose to keep things that way for a long time. But ultimately, little facts started coming out.

The Loved One met him for lunch one day with a friend, who let it slip that they'd shared a joint the previous weekend. She shot the girl this I-told-you-not-to-talk-about-the-pot glare—Adrian hadn't tried weed (he hadn't even had a drink yet), so the Loved One, understandably, had clocked him as an enormous square who would have nothing to do with an occasional pot-smoker. Cringing, she turned her head toward him, but all she saw was his normal face with his normal smile. He stroked her thigh under the table and steered the conversation back to the topic they'd been on before the pot came up.

She probably thought that his deep feelings for her had mastered his disapproval of her drug use. Truth was, by the time she looked over at him, he'd forgotten about the pot comment. She'd never smoked pot at his place, and she obviously didn't want to talk to him about it, so what did it have to do with the Loved One that the Loved One was when the Loved One was around him?

If you see him for long enough, all the stuff that you haven't told Adrian will start to seem like a secret you're keeping from him. It's not, of course. You're just taking advantage of the new you—and welcome to it. So try to keep a better poker face than the Loved One did when something comes out. And don't act like he's your confessor when you decide to share something with him. There's no need.

The sweet girl played the full-on confession game with him a couple of months after the pot reveal. They were making out in the backseat of his car when she mentioned that she'd gone out with her old boyfriend that past week. He said, "Oh, how did that go?" It had gone fine until she'd told the ex-boyfriend she was dating someone else. That's when he pushed her out of his car—don't worry: parked. Before speeding off, he screamed at her out the window, promising to beat up her new boyfriend if he ever found them together.

Adrian stopped feeling her up and rocked her in his arms until her body relaxed. "I'm sorry he did that." Then he snapped his hand back to her boob and started kissing her again. She seemed to take this as some heroic fearlessness on his part. Truth was, he'd forgotten all about the threat by the time he sucked her tongue back out of her mouth.

Since he'd remained unruffled at that much of her story, the Loved One stopped the make-out session again a few minutes later to reveal that her gem of an old boyfriend had hit her a few times while they were going out. That's why she'd broken up with him. Adrian kissed the tears off her face, held her to his chest, and said, "I'm sorry he did that." Then, thinking that maybe a woman who'd just revealed a history of physical abuse might not want to be held tightly, he loosened his grip.

The second she felt her freedom, she squirmed out of his arms, dropped her head into his lap, pulled his cock out of his pants, and gave him the first blowjob he'd ever gotten in a car. That totally drove out of Adrian's mind the whole my-old-boyfriend-beat-me-and-you're-next thing.

9 The Enthusiast didn't have the benefit of knowing not to compliment Adrian when, the Saturday of their first date, she met him at her door with a pitcher of martinis. They spent the evening drinking and drunk in her living room and, in these hours of mostly forgettable conversation, the Enthusiast repeatedly made the mistake of expressing and then reexpressing how much she liked Adrian Colesberry.

Eventually, she must have picked up on his indifference because at the end of the evening the Enthusiast changed to the winning strategy. As she went off to bed, leaving him to sleep on the couch, she took his face in her hands and asked, "Do you know what I am?"

"No. What are you?"

"I'm boy crazy!"

Nothing could have made Adrian happier.

In announcing her boy-craziness, the Enthusiast perfectly made that shift from liking him for who he worked hard to be to adoring him for something he didn't work for at all. You're welcome of course, to find a reason of your own but, if it's true, follow the Enthusiast's lead and tell him you're boy crazy because her instinct with that comment was dead-on.

10 Adrian developed a strong prejudice against a woman talking up her sexual expertise because the only person who'd ever courted him by saying nasty things was the Wife, and she was a complete dud. On the other hand, the Great One and the Kind One never said anything sexual outside of bed, even once he started fucking them, and they proved to be epically magnificent lovers. Pre-sex dirty talk only got promoted from negative to neutral because of one experience he had with one pre-sex dirty talker who did deliver—and how:

On a night out, this girl crushed herself up against Adrian in a crowded bar. They made eye contact. He said, "Excuse me. Hi."

True to form, his "hi" didn't get this girl right away, but hours later, at the end of the evening, she came up to him again and they started talking up a storm. Ten minutes into their conversation, the barkeep announced last call, which sent her into a panic. She said with urgency, "Can I kiss you?" He said yes and they started making out. While getting thrown out of the bar, they exchanged numbers.

On the phone planning their first date, the Expert threw a lot of face cards on the table: She offered up anal sex for one, and, if that wasn't enough, she mentioned that one of her girlfriends, who'd seen him at the bar that night, would happily join them for a two-girl blowjob. She said she'd eat pussy for him too, because even though she was totally straight and not attracted to girls at all, she enjoyed hooking up with girls if it turned a man on.

Then, in a genius move, she seasoned her brothel-menu of available perversions with a dash of modesty: Laughing, the Expert bragged about how many men she would have fucked by the time he picked her up that Friday, then said, "No, seriously, I'm not really sleeping with anyone right now."

In other words, "I'll be a whore for *you*, but I'm not a whore." This is a wonderful message to send Adrian Colesberry.

11 Shortly before they got married, Adrian and the Wife were walking through a crowded shopping mall when, without warning, she jumped up on the wall of a fountain and started singing a show tune from an old musical, belting it out at the top of her lungs, and hijacking the attention of everyone within a fifty-foot radius.

He screwed on a smile for the first half verse, thinking that at any second she would bring the joke to a welcomed end. Only she didn't. The Wife finished the first verse and rounded into the refrain like she was getting an ovation. Only she wasn't. Unable to bear the hate looks from her ambushed audience, Adrian turned and walked slowly away, hoping that she would feel compelled to rejoin the herd.

Tip: *When Adrian deliberately removes himself from your location, it's a sign that he's mortally embarrassed by whatever it is that you're doing.*

No worries if this happens to you; just figure out what you're doing to embarrass him and stop it. That'll quickly return him to your side. The sensitive reader should not imagine that walking away is Adrian's response of first resort. Before up and taking a hike, he employs many subtle signals that your above-average social perception will pick up on right away—avoiding eye contact, nervous laughter, morbid silence, among others.

The Wife never caught on to Adrian's lesser signals, but she did notice the walking away. When she finally caught up with him, she was furious. He said he didn't like singing in public, but she didn't see that as an acceptable personal preference on the order of "I don't like sugar in my coffee." The Wife decided that Adrian's aversion to singing in public was a profound defect in his personality. As a cure, she took to singing at tables in intimate restaurants, in buses, in stores—mostly show tunes, but popular songs too.

In the hopes that she would stop doing it in public, Adrian demonstrated more interest when she sang at home. This home pacification strategy backfired big—she didn't think of their singing in private as a substitute for singing in public but instead saw it as rehearsal time for the big stage that was the party, the restaurant, the clothing store, the movie line, the theater intermission.

Understandably then, Adrian will be a bit twitchy when you go out in public the first few times. He's anxiously examining your behavior for tendencies toward bizarre exhibitionism—body movements that will turn into some unsolicited folk dancing, a rhyming in your speech that might break out into a spontaneous

Beat-poetry recital. Once he realizes that none of this is going to happen, he'll relax.

12 Not knowing about his public behavior jitters created an awkward situation for the Great One. Before he jumped in his car to go home after their first date, she stepped up to kiss him. They made out for just a second, then he started the drive back. His phone rang before he hit the highway. It was the Great One.

> TGO: Did you have a good time?
>
> ADRIAN: Yeah, I had a great time.
>
> TGO: Oh, good. I wasn't sure.
>
> ADRIAN: What?! Why?
>
> TGO: You acted like you didn't want to kiss me.
>
> ADRIAN: Oh, that? I wanted to kiss you! I just . . . I had bad breath.
>
> TGO: I thought you didn't like me.
>
> ADRIAN: No way. I really like you.
>
> TGO: That's a relief! (laughing)
>
> ADRIAN: Yeah.

Totally lame of Adrian to blame it on his breath, which wasn't freshly brushed but certainly wasn't the main reason he didn't want to make out on the street by his car. The main reason he didn't want to make out on the street by his car was that they were out on the street by his car.

"Hang on," the outdoor-sex-loving reader may be saying, "I don't just want to kiss Adrian in public; I want to full-on fuck him in public. If he's got a problem with kissing, how am I going to get what I need?" There is a work-around: Get him drunk.

This method was established not by the Great One but by his first girlfriend after the divorce, the Enthusiast, who consistently turned heads in their direction by making out with Adrian. In the most crowded bar or theater lobby, she'd plop on his lap and start full-on tongue-kissing him, as if they were alone on her couch. This was incredibly embarrassing for him. When offended patrons would catch his eye, he'd return their disapproving glance with a frank look of agreement. If a girl's tongue hadn't been in his mouth, he might have explained, "Yes, this is horribly inappropriate, but I don't care because a girl's tongue is in my mouth."

Even assuming that the Great One knew about the Enthusiast's technique for getting Adrian to have sex in public (and it's imprudent to assume that the Great One didn't know about everything), it would have been criminally irresponsible of her to get Adrian drunk right before sending him on his drive home, so good on her for holding back.

13 When he gets to your snatch, Adrian abandons his back-of-the-finger technique due to its impracticality.

14 On their second date, the Great One found out about Adrian's timing particularities and about the difficulties of adjusting his schedule. The weekend after their first date, she had arranged to be up in his neighborhood, house-sitting just a few blocks from him. They started their Saturday afternoon on her friend's couch. After a couple of hours talking about pretty nearly everything, she asked, "Can we make out?!" She sounded annoyed, like he'd been a tease to let them babble on for so long without making a pass at her. He said "Sure, great!" Then she just attacked him.

It's not that he wasn't ready to roll, but it was only their second date and you know what that means: mouth kissing, touching face with back of fingers, touching hand. Plus, it was two in the afternoon. He wasn't even going to bust out his mega-sensuous back-of-his-fingers face touching until sunset. Make no mistake, Adrian loves fucking in the midafternoon and morning, but until he's fucked you at all, he'll just assume he won't be getting lucky until after dark.

Only, the Great One wanted to get busy while the sun was out, and she succeeded. So, for your education, let's look at how she did it. First, she intuited an important rule: If you are going on a second date with Adrian, he definitely wants to fuck you. He'll throw out his stupid schedule and fuck you right after "Hello." You just have to give him a stronger-than-usual signal. For example, if you start fucking him, Adrian would interpret that as a sign that it's OK for him to fuck you. Alternately, you could start making out with him, or, like the Great One did so brilliantly, you could say that you want to make out with him and then start making out with him.

Adrian's almost unbelievable obtuseness about your green-light signals and the seemingly bizarre back-of-the-fingers touching of your face and breasts can be blamed on his never dating in high school. Teen Adrian is still in there somewhere, not believing that any woman would want his hands or mouth, much less his penis, anywhere near her.

15 The Wife disliked standard foreplay—didn't want him eating her out or even finger-fucking her. So, with his encouragement, she proposed some foreplay substitutes—activities she said would help get her motor running, such as tickling. Unfortunately, his tickling failed to turn her on, so she tickled him, if only to demonstrate proper technique.

He hated being tickled. But with the sex carrot dangling in front of his face, he suffered through with no result.

He took part in many other nonstandard forms of foreplay, from pimple-popping to massage to talking, all the way up to wrestling. He hoped that once they were engaged in some type of naked body contact, he could finesse them into fucking. He couldn't. So ultimately, he stopped playing along.

All of that decoy foreplay has left Adrian suspicious about any activity that doesn't involve a snatch or a cock or both. Although he sincerely wishes that you and he could lie in bed for hours, just holding each other and talking about everything and nothing without fucking having to be a part of it, he can't, and fucking does have to be a part of it—at least at first.

The sexually enthusiastic reader might be protesting, "But I'm not Adrian's ex-wife. I will fuck his brains out. I just want a lot of cuddling up front." See how you and Adrian are so alike: He's not his ex-wife either and he will *cuddle* your brains out. He just wants a lot of *fucking* up front. It's like you two are sides of a leaf or coin.

16 After their third date, Adrian and the Innocent One ended up at her place, drunk. She stripped down to her bra and panties and lay down on her bed. Adrian joined her and they made out for a bit. So far, so good. Then right before he took her panties down, she jumped up and turned all the lights off. He only had the glow from the streetlamps sneaking through the curtains.

Between the dim lighting and the shadow thrown by his head, it was all but impossible for him to see anything. You can imagine how annoying this was, but he didn't object at the time, since he has a strict policy of not complaining to people he's fucking while he's fucking them.

(The strategic reader might see an opportunity to eliminate any complaining Adrian might do period by commencing to fuck him midcomplaint. This could work, but remember that with knowledge comes responsibility: Don't use your knowledge for evil.)

The next time, Adrian volunteered to cut off the lights himself. His tone communicated that he had understood her need for darkness and was eager to oblige her, but this was something of a deception. On getting up, he sneakily struck a compromise between her needs and his by leaving the bathroom light on and the bathroom door ajar. When he moved his head out of the way . . . there she was. Very nice.

17 The traveling-businessman dad of Adrian's best friend from seventh grade had a collection of the hardest, hard-core porn magazines that could be purchased at airport newsstands. Adrian spent the night almost every Saturday, and Sunday mornings he would wake up before the rest of the household, sneak into the dad's office—Adrian's personal porn lending library—and check out a few journals for his studies.

He didn't masturbate while looking at the magazines. No one had yet brought this fine idea to his attention, and even if someone had, he only masturbated in the shower and the logistical difficulties of taking a magazine in there . . . impossible. He studied the photojournalistic layouts, of course, learning from them how to identify the sexually available woman in her various natural habitats—the municipal park, the kitchen, the auto-repair shop, the grocery store produce section, the office, the flower garden, the hippie commune, and the upscale restaurant.

He didn't only look at the pictures, though. After getting to the last of the photographic layouts, Teen Adrian would flip back to read the letters to the editor—his primary source of information about sex, and way better than what he was getting from his only other source: classmates telling him about what they'd read in porn magazines.

Admittedly, most of the things Adrian learned haven't found a practical application in his life. He has never, for instance, been able to put into use all he knows about how to coax a truck-stop waitress into giving up anal sex on her smoke break in the king-size cabin of his big rig.

But his studies were still worth it: When your sexual desires go beyond Adrian's personal experience, rest easy that he has a large knowledge base of pornographic epistolary literature to draw upon.

CHAPTER 3

Oral Sex with Adrian Colesberry

Eating Pussy

Eating pussy is the centerpiece of Adrian Colesberry's sexual game plan.[1] Every time you drop your panties for him, you can expect that he'll go down and stay down until you've either had an obvious orgasm or dragged his face out of your box. Adrian will approach you with a basic strategy, but since every snatch is unique (like a snowflake), that's only a starting point.[2] He'll experiment with different techniques and styles until he finds the combination that you enjoy the most. If you'd like to steepen his learning curve, fill out the table on the next page.

Adrian's Masturbation Theory of Cunnilingus

When exactly to move to the clitoris is the only thing that Adrian finds even slightly tricky about eating pussy. Early on, he developed this theory: If a woman masturbated by fingerwork or with a vibrator, he should go to her clitoris relatively early. If by humping a pillow, he should work the labia and vagina for an extended period of time before making the transition.

One side effect of this theory is that Adrian Colesberry will, pretty early in your relationship, ask how you masturbate. The dubious reader may not buy this business about his only asking so that he can make things better between your thighs. "I'm not about to give him a hard-on by telling him how I masturbate."

But even if that's all he wants, isn't giving Adrian Colesberry a hard-on with a story about how you masturbate enough of a good thing on its own?

Cunnilingus is like a high-end automobile: plenty of options. But not everybody wants her cunnilingus fully loaded: What some find delightful, others find distracting. Take a second to check off your own preferences so that Adrian will know how you like it.

Anything inside the vagina	☐ *No*	☐ *With fingers*	☐ *With toy*
Direct G-spot stimulation	☐ *No*	☐ *With fingers*	☐ *With toy*
Perineal action	☐ *No*	☐ *With mouth*	☐ *With fingers*
Get the asshole involved	☐ *No*	☐ *With mouth*	☐ *With fingers*
Anything inside the asshole	☐ *No*	☐ *With fingers*	☐ *With toy*
Do you want to cum?	☐ *No*	☐ *Yes*	☐ *Depends*
Do you ejaculate or have an interest in ejaculating?	☐ *No*	☐ *Yes*	☐ *Maybe*

If you found in this table some items that you hope Adrian won't try, you're hoping in vain. Regardless of what you checked, he'll try them all. He'd be negligent not to. He doesn't know how you like it best, and maybe you don't either. Be assured that Adrian is very sensitive to the slightest disagreeable sound, interrupted breathing pattern, or sustained muscular stiffness. If you're not on board with anything, he'll notice and cut it out.

The Dilemma of the Cook

For the reader whose tendency would be to skip over all this trial-and-error period by telling Adrian exactly what to do, take a beat and consider following Adrian's rule where it comes to giv-

ing directions in bed: Until you've sampled what's on the menu, don't start ordering the cook around.

Consider this: If you hired a chef and gave them a recipe for your mama's sweet rolls, you might get a good version of your mama's sweet rolls. But what if later you found out that they used to be the head pastry chef for some super-fancy restaurant and they can cook all kinds of mini-tortes and éclairs and multiple layer cakes? Well, wouldn't you feel like an idiot for having instructed this incredibly talented baker to make your mother's sweet rolls for months when you could've been eating like royalty that whole time?

If you ask too soon, you'll never get better than you've gotten.

Cocksucking

Years before anyone had been civil enough to put his penis in her mouth, Adrian had heard and read a lot about the good blowjob—about givers who were exacting in their skill and receivers who demanded a finely crafted fellatio. All this sounded absurd to Adrian. He swore that if a woman ever did that for him, he'd never complain about any part of the transaction. True to his word, he hasn't complained yet and he won't complain to you, either.[3]

One more important note: Adrian won't cum while you're sucking his cock; he will never beg or even ask for head, and far from hoping you'll suck his cock all night long, he won't let you go at it for more than a few minutes before rolling on a condom to fuck you. Upon encountering these behaviors, avoid at all costs the erroneous conclusion that Adrian doesn't like getting his cock sucked. He does.[4]

Enthusiasm

When he eats your box, Adrian is not married to technique but does pour into it all the gratitude and excitement of a teenager who never thought he'd get close to a real-live snatch. As a result, there will be no doubt in your mind that Adrian wants to go down on you. On the other hand, Adrian will have recurring doubts that you want to go down on him, even in the face of evidence to the contrary.[5]

Tip: *Do make a point of communicating to Adrian, verbally if necessary, how much you enjoy sucking him off.*

To understand why you need to articulate your enjoyment more than once, you should know that there's a voice in his head that periodically pops up to tell him, "She doesn't really want to do this. All girls think it's gross. They just do it because they think they have to." With Adrian, since you're not going to make him cum while you're down there, for you the *job* part of the blowjob is mainly to counter that voice in his head.

The 69

Like a virtuoso violinist, Adrian feels that his cunnilingus is best enjoyed as a solo act, unaccompanied by a brass band or a penis in your mouth, respectively. If you're having to donate half your attention to delivering some oral sex of your own, you might miss the new thing he's thought to do with your labia. And that would be a real shame. The converse also applies. When you're sucking his cock, Adrian would like to get the best blowjob you've got in you at that moment, not the one you deliver when he's doing everything he can to distract your clitoris.

Despite these qualifications, there are three reasons that Adrian might opt for the 69.

1. It's good dirty fun.

2. If you want to cum in his mouth and if it takes you a while to cum, Adrian will either switch into the 69 or fuck you occasionally to keep his penis entertained. If that sentence confused you, try it in Boolean:

IF ((cum in mouth) AND (cum>10 mins)) THEN 69 OR fucking

Clearer?

3. You are not sucking his cock enough or at all, and he switches into the 69 to give you a hint.[6] The fact that the 69 can be used as a referendum on your generosity toward his cock might make the considerate reader nervous when Adrian flips into it. "How can I tell the difference between his dirty-fun 69 position and his hint-hint 69?" In all honesty, you can't. If anything makes you wonder, "Am I paying enough attention to Adrian's cock with my hands and mouth?" don't look to Adrian, look inside your own heart.

Smothering

Nearly everyone Adrian's been with has sat on his face at one time or another, but none of them have been super into it, so Adrian has limited experience in this area. Left to his own devices, he'll only flip you into this position as a dirty variation, since he feels like he does his best work when you're on your back. But needless to say, if you prefer sitting on his face, that's what you'll be doing. He's done it enough to know that you need to take responsibility for his access to air. Also, if you really go to town grinding around, you'll need to mind his nose, which could be easily crushed by your pubic bone. Adrian isn't super turned on by oxygen deprivation but he does like a snatch in his face, so you're in pretty safe territory.

Skull-Fucking

The sensitive reader may be worrying, "Skull-fucking?! That sounds like I can be giving Adrian a generous, nuanced blowjob when, without warning, he'll start trying to feed his cock past my tonsils!"

That's not at all how it works, of course. Your misconstrual can be blamed on the marketing flunky who coined the term "skull-fucking." Once you hear what it is, you'll probably realize that you've been doing it for years: Skull-fucking is to fellatio what smothering is to cunnilingus. It's a blowjob with a difference in who does the work. In a blowjob, the giver moves her mouth around the penis; in skull-fucking, the person with the penis does the work of moving it in and out of the other person's mouth. That's all. Couldn't be simpler.

Why would Adrian want to do this? Well, as much good press as the blowjob gets and deserves, most of the time Adrian just needs something to fuck.[7] Therefore, occasionally, while you're giving him a blowjob, he'll start fucking your mouth. No gagging you, no attempted deep-throating. During your previous episodes of fellatio, he'll have noticed how far you take his penis inside your mouth and he'll only push in that far.

Deep-Throating

Adrian does not expect you to be able to take his erect penis down your throat. He views sword swallowing as more of a circus trick than an essential sexual skill and will certainly find your particular method of orally pleasuring him to be transcendently magnificent, with or without this element.

At the same time, the reader who proudly practices the art of deep-throating shouldn't interpret Adrian's laissez-faire attitude as indifference. Hardly. Be assured that this particular circus trick will marvelously impress and delight him.[8]

1   From its central role in his sexual game plan, you'd think that Adrian's career in eating snatch had a promising beginning. It didn't; anything but. The first girl he went down on was, naturally enough, the First One. As he headed between her legs for the only time, she said, "You can try it, but you won't like it." Some bad experience with an early boyfriend who thought it was yicky or something—he never got the details.

But as Adrian had read many favorable accounts, no warning, however well-intentioned, was going to stop him from trying it out. After a few licks, he drew his head back because, as you could have predicted, he wanted to get his first extreme close-up view of his first real-live snatch. On seeing him pull away, the First One assumed that he was recoiling in disgust, and immediately dragged him up, saying, "I told you you wouldn't like it." She obviously wasn't interested in getting head, so he just dropped it.

2   The Loved One, his second college girlfriend, was the first girl Adrian got to know face-to-snatch. She came in his mouth the very first time—and he had no technique at all yet, just enthusiasm for the project, which is the most important thing anyway. As her climax approached, she squeezed his head between her thighs until he saw stars. Down the road, he figured out how to position his head so that her scissor-thighs wouldn't hurt his brain so much, but that first time, she caught him right between the temples.

Mighty-thighed reader, Adrian realizes that your cracking his skull like a nut upon achieving your orgasm isn't an ill-meaning assault against his person but rather a flattering review of his pussy-eating skills. As much as he appreciates your appreciating him, do give him either a warning or a crash helmet.

The Loved One's clitoris was supersensitive so, with his encouragement, she showed him a licking pattern that made an upside-down V in that groove between her inner and outer labia—grazing her hood without hammering right on her clitoris. Once she neared her orgasm, she'd have him turn all his attention to her clitoris and that's when her leg-scissor thing would happen. Out of habit, he'll start off with this but if you like something different, do follow the Loved One's example and give Adrian a tour of your snatch.

After gaining a comfort level with the basics, he got super-experimental with the Loved One—he gave her rimjobs while he finger-fucked her snatch; he finger-fucked her asshole while he ate her snatch. . . . Pretty nearly everything that Adrian does while eating pussy today, he beta tested between those thighs. This includes a maneuver that he never quite perfected where he'd nuzzle her clitoris with his nose while tongue-fucking her. If you're interested in this nose-rubbing technique, kindly inform Adrian Colesberry, and he'll be happy to throw it back into development.

3 Knowing Adrian's no-complaint policy, it won't intimidate you to learn that the First One gave a great blowjob. He knew this because one day she said to him, "I give a great blowjob." She didn't say it boastfully but just put it out there as some information he might find interesting. And he did, very.

He had no idea what a blowjob was supposed to be like in the first place, so his scientifically educated mind was thrilled to get ahold of a cocksucking standard that he could use to evaluate all his future cocksucking experiences.

If you are proud of an aspect of your sexual performance, feel free to point it out to Adrian Colesberry so he won't fail to notice in the confusion of passion. Maybe you give an enormously entertaining handjob or have exquisitely well-controlled vaginal muscles. Do mention it so he can commend you on your skill, as he did with the First One.

A few seconds after dropping this knowledge on him, the First One started giving him one of her Great Blowjobs and, for his continuing education, narrated her performance in step-by-step detail. For the record, here's how she sucked cock:

Before starting, she pushed her tongue over her bottom front teeth and curled her top lip inward to cover her uppers. Then she placed his head inside the flesh funnel that she'd made of her mouth and clamped his shaft in her fist. She was careful to press the webbing of her thumb right against her bottom lip so there wouldn't even be an air gap between her hand and her mouth. Once satisfied with the structural integrity of her mouth-hand-combination skin-sleeve, she started jacking him off by moving her arm in step with her head.

After a minute of this, she broke away to state the obvious, "See, this way, my teeth never touch you."

Unless it's a trick you've already got down, don't worry about getting your teeth out of the way for Adrian Colesberry. In his later experiences, he found out that it was kind of stimulating for his cock to slide against a few ivories. What will turn him on about your giving him a blowjob is less the isolated sensation than the nastiness of your actually putting his penis in your mouth. And while he's not inviting you to chew on it, nothing tells him his cock is in your mouth like crashing into a molar now and again.

In that moment, however, Adrian knew what the First One wanted to hear, so he enthused, "Oh yeah! Feels like you don't have any teeth at all!" Finally satisfied that he understood how great her Great Blowjobs really were, she got back to sucking his cock with no more interruptions. He learned later that she'd been painstakingly trained in the method of the Great Blowjob by an early boyfriend—one who obviously suffered from a clinically diagnosable paranoia about getting his dick bit off.

The technique did manage to transform her hands and mouth into an uncanny simulation of her vagina. But that seemed pointless since she already had a for-real vagina two feet south, one that Adrian's penis had free access to. Would you build a scale model of Stonehenge two barley fields away from Stonehenge? Obviously not.

To the reader who has perfected the Great Blowjob, you may feel as if Adrian's indifference has removed the straightest and strongest arrow from your quiver. Don't panic. He will love whatever technique you practice, as long as it involves your inviting Adrian's penis into your mouth.

Regardless of how much he wowed about the Great Blowjob, because he never came in her mouth, she never believed he liked it. A real pity since the First One performed the Great Blowjob with such skill. She's surely still out there today, regularly oral-ejaculating some lucky guy. Cheers to you, sir!

For Adrian's liking, there was just too much method and not enough passion in her focus on her tongue angle and her hand position. He didn't want her to blow him to make him cum. He wanted her to blow him because she needed his cock in her mouth more than she needed to breathe. As it turned out, he would have to wait a long time for that. He would have to wait for the Great One.

Paradoxically, the Great One did not give a Great Blowjob. Her cocksucking didn't fall into any pattern that he could detect. He certainly couldn't accuse her of having a technique. She just had passion. She sucked his cock with her whole person. Her tits and face and neck and hair—they weren't just body parts for him to fondle but sense organs of her own to fondle him with.

4   If it seems ridiculous that someone would come to the conclusion that Adrian didn't like a blowjob, know that the concern is drawn from his own true history.

Right before relieving him of his virginity, the First One had given him a little head, but she didn't suck his cock any more after that. He never said anything about it, thinking that maybe she'd just sucked him off that once as an introductory bonus.

Then a couple of months in, she mentioned that he was the first man she'd been with who didn't like head. He was all, "Who said I didn't like head?! I love head! Where's the line for head? And why am I not standing in it?!"

She explained that he'd tensed up that first time, so she'd figured he didn't like it. He responded that if he had tensed up, it was from pure amazement that a woman was actually putting his penis in her mouth. She immediately adjusted her behavior in light of the new information. From that conversation forward, she regularly gave him the Great Blowjob. Point is, he spent months wanting head and not getting head even though the First One herself had put head on the menu from the get-go.

The forward-speaking reader might wonder, "Adrian, if you wanted your cock sucked so bad, why didn't you just ask for it?" Good question. The answer: He's terrible at communicating what he wants. Always has been. Won't be asking you, either.

5   Though it seems impossible, Adrian even had doubts that the Great One wanted to suck his cock. These doubts came to the fore the first time she got her period. With pussy licking and finger-banging off the menu, he massaged her back and played with her boobs and she sucked his cock. Then she sucked his cock some more. And after that, she sucked his cock.

It made him self-conscious—getting all the pleasure and not giving any, but when he said so out loud, the Great One dropped him out of her mouth and laughed. "Who said you were the only one getting pleasure from it?" Adrian felt so stupid. He'd given her head for ages the weekend before. Why couldn't she like sucking cock just as much as he liked eating pussy? She could of course and that ended that, but for her only. You'll have to end his concerns regarding you.

6 Adrian first tried the entirely unsubtle but effective 69-as-request-for-a-blowjob back in college with the Loved One. Her previous boyfriend had popped her cherry for her. But judging from her extreme, virginlike tightness, the guy had done very little of the follow-up work required to break in her box. It took twenty minutes of cunnilingus for her to be able to fuck comfortably for five. After learning that she'd spent over a year with the guy, he came to the conclusion that she must've sucked him off most of the time.

This and later evidence of her know-how in the blowjob department made it even stranger that, after being together for a month, the Loved One hadn't gotten her mouth anywhere near his cock. It didn't bother him; he just figured, "When she wants to suck my cock, she'll suck it." But his figuring didn't pan out half quick enough for his liking, so one day, he decided to give her a little hint by going down on her in the 69 position.

To avoid being thought ungenerous, the reader might want to know what exactly "quick enough" means to Adrian Colesberry. As a general rule of thumb, if he's gone down on you a dozen times, it's a good idea to give back a bit. He's not counting, and he's not tracking his time eating your snatch against your time cocksucking. He just wants to occasionally feel the love that is your putting his cock in your mouth. That's all.

Adrian didn't straddle the Loved One's head and poke her in the eye with his cock. That first time using the 69 technique, he just maneuvered her onto her side and casually laid his erection on the mattress near her face, not so close as to be ungentlemanly, but not so far that she'd have to do much more than turn her head to fetch it into her mouth.

She took the hint immediately and started sucking away. From then on, whenever he wanted head, he just flipped into a 69 position, and it was done. A few weeks of that business was all it took for her to initiate cocksucking on her own. One day, he'd just finished eating her out and was fixing to roll on a condom when she pushed him onto his back and took him into her mouth. Success!

7 Adrian's skull-fucking career started off quite naturally: As you'll find out, one of his favorite things is to swap off between going down on you and fucking you. In his mind, it geometrically increases your pleasure, not knowing how he'll be pleasuring you next. The Great One certainly enjoyed it, so much that she felt obliged to explain why she wasn't returning the favor in kind: She said she'd be only too happy to blow him between bouts of fucking but for a particular aversion she had for the taste of the latex condoms they were using.

He understood and said he just enjoyed swapping off without expecting her to do the same. But the next time she went down on him, their talking about it left him wanting to fuck something, anything, so he reflexively started pushing his cock in and out of her mouth.

As soon as he noticed what he was doing, not only did he stop moving his cock but froze up his whole body.*

The instant that he stopped, the Great One made nonsense of his overcaution. She hadn't been scared off at all by his fucking her mouth. She acted like his cock was a toy that they were sharing. He'd wanted to play with it, so she'd let him fuck her mouth. When he stopped, she figured that he was giving it back to her so she could play with it for a while. And that's how skull-fucking became part of their repertoire.

8   Only one woman in the pantheon ever deep-throated Adrian. It was the Expert, and for future generations, a few words should be said about her blowjobs because her overall technique, leaving aside the entertaining deep-throat trick she had mastered, was both economic and effective.

For each minute she spent sucking his cock, his penis spent only fifteen seconds in her mouth. She would swallow his entire cock into her throat to start, but after that she'd just give him a

---

* It has been said before but cannot be emphasized enough that any awkwardness he displays during this act should not be interpreted as Adrian's not liking a blowjob. Occasionally he will become self-conscious about his penis being in your mouth and revert to Teen Adrian's worry that if he ever moved while a woman was sucking him off, he'd scare her away.

Grown-up Adrian realizes this is ridiculous. He has read plenty of field guides and knows that cocksuckers aren't particularly skittery. But until his panic passes, he'll minimize his intrusion into your environment, breathing slowly and regularly and, if he has to rearrange his body for comfort, he'll shift in stages, avoiding any sudden movement that might make you disengage your mouth from his penis.

handjob. She kept her open mouth right there and checked back in with the deep-throat trick occasionally, just to sell the whole thing as a blowjob, but it barely was. Adrian didn't complain, mind you; her handjob was one of the best blowjobs he'd ever gotten.

Tip: *The reader whose mouth gets tired sucking Adrian's cock should take a tip from the Expert's technique and rely more on hand action than mouth action.*

CHAPTER 4

Fucking Adrian Colesberry

Positions

Historically, Adrian has spent 85 percent of his time in mission-ary, 5 percent in doggie-style, 5 percent in woman-on-top, and 5 percent in all others combined. It might interest you that he has only ever cum in missionary. This could be seen as a justification for his camping out there all the time, but a little critical thinking should make you wonder if he camps out in missionary because it's the only place he can cum or if he only cums there because it's the position he camps out in all the time. In any case, don't imag-ine that making love to Adrian Colesberry consists of a little fore-play followed by a measure of spirited pussy-eating then a polite request for you to lie on your back so that he can ejaculate.

He has proven himself more than willing to experiment with different positions over the years. He enjoys some more, some less, based on the following six criteria:

1. Comfort, including exhaustion. If the position hurts, he won't like it for long. A position that seems comfortable at the first thrust may, after some time, begin to overtax a muscle. This can even happen in his beloved missionary position.
2. Gravity on downstroke. Adrian gets off on thrusting into a woman, like he's trying to fuck his way back into the womb.

So he will fuck more vigorously in any position where he's on top.

3. Body contact. Maximum body contact is important. If one or both of you can put your arms and legs around the other, so much the better. Although when it's hot, body contact can become something of a negative. (All the rankings below assume a comfortable ambient temperature.)

4. Range of motion. Adrian vastly prefers for his penis to be all but in the air at the top of his stroke and buried at the bottom. Any position that uses only part of this range of motion is inferior.

5. Scenery. Nothing beats looking at a woman's face, if only to check out her changes in expression. Her ass runs a tight second.

6. Access. The ability to kiss a woman during sex is important to Adrian, as is his ability to touch her fun parts.

The alert reader will have noticed that Adrian Colesberry cannot satisfy all of his preferences at the same time. The following table and graph illustrate the tradeoffs involved among the various positions, where 1 is the worst and 5 is the best.

POSITION	COMFORT	GRAVITY	BODY CONTACT	RANGE OF MOTION	SCENERY	ACCESS	OVERALL
Missionary	4	5	5	5	4	1	24
Doggie-Style	3	3	1	4	4	5	20
Lazy Dog[1]	5	5	5	4	2	1	22
Woman-on-Top[2]	5	1	3	1	5	3	18
From the Side, Spooning	4	3	5	2	1	4	19
Lazy Couch Arm[3]	5	3	1	5	4	4	22

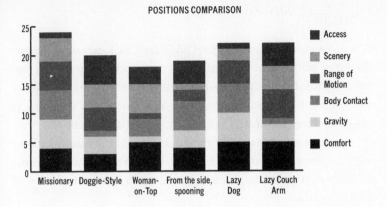

POSITIONS COMPARISON

Legend:
- Access
- Scenery
- Range of Motion
- Body Contact
- Gravity
- Comfort

Categories: Missionary, Doggie-Style, Woman-on-Top, From the side, spooning, Lazy Dog, Lazy Couch Arm

Changing Positions

When performed with suitable vigor, fucking involves a lot of shifting around. You and Adrian can choose to navigate through position changes like the hero and heroine of a Victorian novel: "Would you mind terribly flipping into female superior?" rejoined with, "My pleasure!" followed by limbs being politely rearranged with an occasional, "Why, excuse me!" until the desired posture is attained and Adrian has completely lost his erection because his vast preference is to manhandle you into a position change.[4] What he's trying to say with his physicality is, "You're getting fucked this way whether you like it or not." (Unless you don't like it, in which case he'll change positions immediately.)

So when Adrian pushes your thighs farther apart, it's not because you didn't throw them wide enough in the first place, he just wants to have had a part in winging them open. And don't be offended if, after conscientiously arranging yourself on knees and elbows, he hauls your hips into place. He's not criticizing your original posture. He just wants your ass to be where he put it.

Lubrication

When you start fucking Adrian Colesberry, he'll rely on foreplay alone for lubrication—enough head, and everything should be good to go. If the row gets stony, he'll drop down to clear the furrow, then get back behind the plow. Needless to say, give him a heads-up if you feel things drying out, but most likely he'll be the one to notice. As sexperts are perhaps too fond of reminding men, there are few nerves inside the vagina, so even with a condom on, the body part most likely to detect a change in friction is the tip of Adrian's penis.

Don't imagine, from this description, that Adrian plans to 100 percent spit-lubricate your lovemaking or that it's the only reason he's going down on you. If that's the way you cum, he's hoping to help you do that of course, but mainly he's aiming to make your levels of arousal more or less equal by the time he pushes his cock inside you.

If the need for personal lubrication arises, Adrian will have some on hand. If you don't mind, he'd just as soon stay away from the flavored varieties because the beginning of fucking doesn't mean the end of eating your box, and Adrian doesn't want any synthetic flavorings in the mix.

He's also not into any of the sugary stuff, flavored or not, as it ultimately gets too sticky. He'll have on hand at least one nonsugary, nonflavored water-based lube and a silicone lube for you to choose from. These initial preferences aside, do make it known if you have a personal favorite, and he'll go fetch it.[5]

The ultrafeminine reader may well be balking at all this talk about lube. "I don't know about other ladies, but I'm as wet as rain so won't be needing any of this." Perhaps, but the need for lube isn't about your having insufficient lubrication in general, it's about filling the gaps in the nonoverlapping sections of Adrian's hardness cycle and your wetness cycle.

Adrian doesn't get hard and stay hard. He gets hard, fucks for a bit, then backs off, then gets hard again and in between, his erection isn't in good enough shape to fuck. In his experience, women are no different. A woman gets wet then backs off then gets wet again. Only the two cycles aren't exactly overlapping but offset, as illustrated in the Hardness/Wetness Cycle Comparison graph.

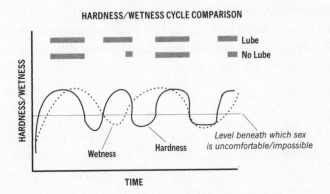

HARDNESS/WETNESS CYCLE COMPARISON

The solid line is Adrian's hardness level. The dashed line is a woman's wetness level. When the sinusoidal arousal curves dip below the midline, either Adrian isn't hard enough or she isn't wet enough and sex becomes either impossible or uncomfortable. As the curves offset, they are not always above the line at the same time. Sometimes the woman is wet enough but Adrian isn't hard and at other times, he is hard enough, but she isn't wet. In that latter case, where he's hard but she's not wet enough, lube comes in to make things comfortable and/or possible. Look at the top bars to see how. The gains may look modest to the naked eye, but in this example lube increases their time at intercourse by 42 percent.

The equality-oriented reader might see an imbalance in this solution. "There's a fix that lets Adrian fuck when I'm not wet enough, where's the fix that I can use when I'm wet but Adrian isn't hard enough?" That's called a dildo. And yes, Adrian would be happy to fuck you with a dildo while his penis is resting—very happy. Thanks for asking. He'll be relieved not to be the first one to bring it up for once.

Talking and Fucking

Adrian welcomes open communication in all aspects of his life. And while fucking isn't the time for a full-on conversation, there are certain things that Adrian says and would welcome hearing you say in the act.

Signals of Appreciation

Adrian will make sounds to communicate his enjoyment. These sounds will be occasional, never turning into an unbroken flow of words and exclamations. In turn, he welcomes any sounds of appreciation you might make. If you pay attention, you'll notice that you are always making more noise than he is. This is no accident: He modulates his own output to be approximately one-third of yours. (If you don't make any noise, he'll breathe softer.)

When you treat Adrian to a handjob or blowjob, he'll give you positive feedback and encouragement by making sounds or statements like, "Oh, that's nice." Interestingly, he won't as often compliment your vagina. Adrian will spend a large portion of his time in bed flat-out worshiping your hole, so it's not that he doesn't appreciate it. In his way of thinking, the fact that your vagina feels good is something that it *is* more than something that it *does,* and he has a working-class prejudice toward doing over being. He's not alone in this bias: Head is called a blow*job* and manual stimulation a hand*job,* but nobody calls fucking a vaginajob.

He does count lubrication as work of a sort, so when he feels you getting wetter, he will provide a "There you are," or a "Good girl," or sometimes even an on-the-nose "You are so wet."

Name Calling

Don't say his name. He's not paranoid that you don't know his name and he won't be impressed that you've remembered it. On hearing you say his name, he's most likely to think you want something, like a glass of water.

If you want him to say your name, he will, but it's not his favorite. Adrian reserves your name for situations when he's getting your attention or he's looking for you in a mall. If Adrian is pinning you to the mattress with his cock, he has found you and he will take it for granted that he has your attention.

Announcing Orgasms

Adrian isn't a fan of calling out his orgasms, as in "I'm cumming!" or "Here it is!" or "Brace yourself!" He's actually managed to stifle orgasms by saying things like that. He hears "I'm cumming" not as, "If you were meaning to give me pleasure, congratulations, you are about to receive the ultimate proof of your success!" He hears it more as, "All stand! His Highness has entered the drawing room." Adrian's sense of humility cannot tolerate even a shadow of this meaning. Hypocritically enough, he'd love to hear the news that you are cumming.

Giving and Taking Direction

It's clear from your commitment to learning how to make love to Adrian Colesberry that you want to be good at it. To this end, you may be looking forward to some on-the-spot pointers from the man himself or even a full-on training session where you learn to give him the perfect handjob, blowjob, whateverjob. This is not going to happen.[6]

Adrian will direct your activities a bit, but he's not going to focus on it unless getting ordered around is your bag. He certainly wouldn't enjoy the reverse: your telling him what to do blow by blow. Instructional comments back and forth are welcomed, needless to say: "speed up," "slow down," "right there," "pinch my nipples," "not yet." And he'll give general hints, such as, "Jerk me off while you do that." But he's going nowhere near "Shape your fingers into the 'OK' gesture and lightly work the shaft at a rate of approximately forty-two strokes per minute."

If you're one of those people for whom quality is job one, Adrian's reluctance to give detailed instructions might seem unacceptable. "If he won't tell me how to do things, how do I know I'm doing them right?" The best way to get things right is to borrow the technique of an optometrist giving an eye exam: "Is this better, or this?" "Do you like it when I work your balls, or no?" "This is me working your balls . . . here it is without. Which do you like better?" He'll appreciate that approach and will do the same for you.

Many times, Adrian will save this evaluative talk for just after, as in, "Did you like that thing I did with your nipples, or was it distracting?" This gives you a way to tell him to cut something out or keep something up without hurting his ego, so do take advantage of it.

Most importantly, keep in mind that when Adrian Colesberry asks you for a sexual favor or tries to tell you how to make things better for him in bed, it might not seem like a big deal to you, but it is a big deal for him.[7] When he asks, "Could you jerk me off while I do this?" he's not hedonistically fine-tuning his sensual inputs to optimize that particular moment of that singular sexual encounter. What he's saying is, "Could you jerk me off while I do this because I hope to be doing this next week and the week after that, so you might want to know that, in general, while I'm doing this, I'd like you to jerk me off."

Dirty Talk

Adrian is happy to pepper your lovemaking with provocative statements in the areas of ordering you to do what you are already doing, asking you if you like what he's already doing to you, and making comments implying that you are nasty for fucking him in the way you are currently fucking him.[8]

He's only chatting it up to turn the both of you on. If anything he says is achieving the opposite effect, do give him a heads-up and he'll put a cork in it. This is a two-way street, by the by. He'd enjoy hearing a sprinkling of these comments from you as well.

Top Dirty-Talk Phrases

The following presents a greatest hits of Adrian's fully developed dirty-talk repertoire, complete with instructions for use. Feel free to borrow from it, and definitely expect to have some of these phrases coming at you when Adrian starts dirty-talking.[9]

- "Does that make you feel dirty?!" Not at all a question but pronounced with a dead certainty that it absolutely does make you feel dirty. He'll sometimes follow this up by answering, "Yeah, you're dirty!"
- "Are you a naughty girl?!" Again, he'll immediately follow up with, "Yeah, you're a naughty girl!" Or sometimes, he'll start with, "You like that?!" kind of like he's noticing for the first time some new aspect of your naughtiness. Then, as if it has made him angry, he'll say, "You're a naughty girl!"
- "You just want to suck my cock all night, don't you?" After changing the words to match your personal anatomy, definitely borrow this one. You know you can't lose there—Adrian does want to eat your box all night long. That's what he showed up for. Do be careful to save this dirty talk for when Adrian is actually eating your box. If you blurt it out while fucking, he might think you want him to stop fucking you and eat your box instead when really you were totally into the fucking and just trotting out a little dirty talk. Yes, it gets tricky. You have to pay attention if you're going to try this stuff.
- And finally—the jewel in Adrian's dirty-talk crown: "Oh, you like it when I treat you like a dirty whore, don't you?!"

Notice how none of these questions have legitimate answers. Nothing about sex makes you feel dirty, much less like a prostitute, and no way would you want to give Adrian head for an entire evening—not even *he* would want that; the entire idea is just stupid.

Sexual Terminology

Despite his comfort with dirty talk, Adrian can still get tripped up by off-putting terminology. Find below a guide to his most and least favorite terms:

The sacred word is certainly his favorite word for the lady parts. The other acceptable synonyms, as you already know from the vocabulary used in these pages, are snatch, hole, box, and pussy (the last mainly in reference to oral sex). The names Adrian can't hear without cringing are the ones that make the lady parts sound unhealthy, such as gash; any of the clearly comical ones, which won't be listed here (but you know who you are, hairy taco); and the ones that go out of their way to make the lady parts seem cutesy, such as clitty for clitoris or poonie or koochie. There's no need for a word that makes the lady parts sound cute. If there were room for only one cute thing in the entire universe, lady parts already would be it.

As far as boy parts, cock is the best by a mile. Dick comes in a distant second. Penis is safe, as are all legitimate anatomical terms for any part. Hard-on works. Tool is OK in a pinch. Euphemisms such as member, love-muscle, and all just turn him off.

As a last note, he really doesn't like the acronym BJ. If you announced, "I'm going to give you a BJ you'll never forget," he would certainly never forget your generous blowjob but would instantly try to forget that you called it a BJ.

Turning On Adrian Colesberry

This topic may seem quite out of order, coming at the end of the chapter on fucking. You'd be right to wonder, "Wouldn't I have turned Adrian on before this?" Yes, of course you would have. But that was on the easy side of fucking. Up front, all you have to do is smile or walk away from him or touch him . . . anywhere—no special knowledge or pro tips required. But say you've gone at it for a while, and he's ready for a rest while you still want some more. That's when it can be more challenging. Here are some things you can do to re-up Adrian's enthusiasm for the project:

1. Let Adrian smack you on the ass.

This particular suggestion doesn't have to do with flipping over in bed at the moment when you sense that he's flagging and having him smack you on the ass (a wonderful idea by itself that deserves and will get its own hearing). It has to do with letting him smack your ass in general. You might be interested to know that Adrian gets the urge to smack your ass all the time: while fucking, of course, but outside the bedroom too—on walks, at the museum, climbing behind you up a flight of stairs, when you bend over to reach across a counter . . . really pretty much any time your ass appears in his field of vision.[10]

The cautious reader might worry that letting Adrian Colesberry smack you on the ass will be the first step on the path to matching master/slave T-shirts; that you'll wake up one morning with a ball gag in your mouth. No such thing. Adrian does not hear your accepting his smack as a general invitation to confuse your pain with your pleasure. It's not a mock punishment or an attempt to cause you discomfort.

Adrian smacks you on the ass as an expression of ownership. His smack says, "That's mine." And if you want him to get turned on by your ass, you do want him to think that he owns it. Not owns it like he'd sell it, but like he has a stake in it. Here's how this pays off in bed: If you get him to invest in your ass by letting him smack it every once in a while, all you have to do to get his interest back up is flop onto your belly and show him what's his. Hand a man the keys to his car and what is he going to do but drive it? Same with Adrian Colesberry and your ass.

2. Masturbate for him.

There's nothing more beautiful to Adrian than a woman masturbating—no natural wonder, no baby kitty, no work of art. You can guess, then, that Adrian would like you to masturbate for him. The accommodating reader needn't wait for Adrian to ask. There's no tricky timing involved, like taking a soufflé out of the oven. You can masturbate before he starts fucking you, while he's fucking you, after he's finished fucking you . . . The most convenient moments to masturbate are in those spaces when you're on a natural break, like when he's pulled out to apply lubricant or to check that the condom is still hanging tough. (Safety first!)

There is one thing: If you wouldn't mind, masturbate with your fingers or a toy. That turns him on more than watching you hump a pillow or a rolled-up towel. The pillow-humping reader might be complaining, "But that's just the way I masturbate. Can't he deal with that?" Yes, he can. If you're trying to get yourself off, Adrian's happy to watch you or help you in whatever way. He'll lie there while you hump his leg; he'll hold a tissue to your nose if you get off by sneezing. Whatever.

But when you're masturbating to turn him on, use your hands. It might help to think about it less as masturbation and more as fucking yourself. Just by making slow circles around your clitoris, you're leading by example: "Look, I'm fucking myself, I wonder if anyone wants to join in?" Yes, someone does want to join in. That someone is Adrian Colesberry.

3. Have Adrian finger-bang your asshole.

(See Chapter 6.)

4. Have Adrian give you a full-on spanking.

(As opposed to a one-off smack, see Chapter 7.)

5. Want him.

The most reenergizing aphrodisiac in the world is being wanted.
The accommodating reader might wonder, "What about my being
naked on a bed with my legs flung open does not communicate to
Adrian that I want him?" Certainly, this is enough. But in a relationship where you are regularly being wanted by and wanting the
other person, there is the need for heroic expressions of desire.
There are a million ways to make Adrian feel especially wanted,
clothes off or on. No special instructions apply. It's up to you and
your imagination to pull this off.[11]

Have a Moist Towelette

You've heard the question "How do you know when you're finished making love?" That question is easily answered with Adrian
Colesberry because he has an ending ritual: When you're finished,
he'll roll off you, pop out of bed, start running the hot water in the
bathroom, bring you a glass of cold water from the kitchen, chat
for a bit while you sip it, return to the bathroom, wet two washcloths in the now-hot water, and wring them out. Warm, moist
washcloths in hand, he'll come back to bed, trade you the glass for
one of the washcloths, then, when you're done cleaning off with
it, he'll cup the other one against you until the heat has gone.[12]

1   On his second weekend with the Great One, wouldn't you know that Adrian got a cold sore on his lip. Yes, he gets cold sores. On the mostly well-paved path of learning how to make love to Adrian Colesberry, there are a few potholes.

He tried to fuck her in missionary, but it drove him crazy—her mouth right there but off-limits, so more out of frustration than anything else, Adrian flipped her over flat on her stomach, put a pillow under her hips, leaned his palms on her shoulder blades, and fucked her from behind—like doggie-style except she was flat on the mattress (thus Lazy Dog) and he was holding himself in missionary.

He was so entertained by the position that he stayed there all afternoon. When he rolled off for the last time, the Great One waited a beat and then said she'd enjoyed the fucking from behind a lot and would be happy to fuck that way exclusively, if that's how Adrian had to do it, but that next time they might try missionary or woman-on-top.[*]

---

[*] *The way that the Great One criticized Adrian's lovemaking, that was art. She could have crushed him like a potato chip with a flippant "It's not going to be that from-behind business every time, is it?" But she managed to get across that content while carefully preserving his ego. Here's a breakdown of how she went about it, not only for your benefit but also for the benefit of generations to come:*

THE GREAT ONE'S EXAMPLE	STEPWISE INSTRUCTIONS
"I enjoyed the fucking from behind a lot . . ."	**Step 1.** *What you just did left me completely sexually satisfied.*
". . . and would be happy to fuck that way exclusively, if that's how you have to do it,"	**Step 2.** *If that's all we ever do, good by me.*
". . . but maybe next time we could try missionary or woman-on-top."	**Step 3.** *Here's a suggestion for making things even better.*

Who would not respond positively to this loving, generous method of criticism? You can be sure that Adrian took notes. If he ever has the opportunity to fine-tune some element of your lovemaking, he'll be working right from this script. Here for instance, is what he would say to you if you manhandled his sensitive testicles:

> "I certainly enjoyed the way you treated my testicles like they were ball bearings in a burlap sack. If that's what turns you on, I look forward to your all but popping them out of my scrotum every time we make love, but if it's OK, maybe next time you could try varying the sensation by treating them like they were two small, sensitive glands that, by some cosmic design flaw, are hanging outside of my body."

Adrian immediately realized what had happened: They'd had sex only the once before, and that time his penis hadn't worked so well. As far as the Great One knew, the only way Adrian Colesberry could get it up was to fuck her from behind in Lazy Dog.

Adrian cleared that up right away by explaining that he'd only turned her onto her stomach in the first place because he couldn't kiss her on account of his enormous cold sore. That made her feel *a lot* better. He assured her that he vastly preferred missionary and would be happy to let her ride on top whenever she felt like it.

2 Left to his own devices, Adrian will only use woman-on-top (aka female superior) for taking breaks between bouts of missionary or some other energy-intensive position. Having said that, if you need to grind around to find your orgasm, knock yourself out. Take care not to break his penis, though. The Wife did that to him once, and it really hurt. (It figures that the woman with the least interest in his penis would be the only one to do it any damage.)

But even beyond that one extremely negative experience, the women in his life just haven't been able to generate a large enough range of motion to keep his interest, where "interest" means "hard-on."

Adrian discussed his attitude about female superior with the Great One, minus the harrowing story of his penis breaking—no need to assault her tender sensibilities. After hearing him out, she responded, "Range of motion, huh? We'll work on that."

As he'd promised, Adrian incorporated more woman-on-top into their repertoire, and found that he liked the position a lot more than he thought he did. The Great One's tits hung right in his face, looking twice as big as they did when he was on top. Having no weight to bear with his hands, he took to fondling her boobs. And he had more time just to look at her. She was lovely. Keeping her promise, the Great One worked on her range of motion, to good effect.

3 Freshly showered after an evening of lovemaking, Adrian sat beside the Great One on her couch. Almost immediately he realized that he wanted to fuck her again, but he was too lazy to move them into the bedroom. So after some making out he dragged her ass over the low couch arm and, his feet on the ground, fucked her there (thus Lazy Couch Arm). The Great One gave the position a good review, so Adrian returned to it often when they happened to be in her living room.

4 The Great One, accommodating to a fault, was nearly impossible to manhandle into position changes, as Adrian prefers. From the first hints of his movement, she'd accurately anticipate that he wanted her, say, on her side, and cooperatively shift her hips into place. Without saying the words, she was playing the ultracompliant Victorian novel heroine. He couldn't put his finger on it at the time, but Adrian would have liked a little pushback.

He found the resistance he wanted with his next lover, the Kind One. If he started to move her leg or arm, she'd ask, "What?!" in a kind of annoyed tone.

Forced to explain, he'd say (in an equally annoyed tone), "I want you on your stomach."

And even once she'd understood the move, she'd complain, "OK! OK!" and still not help very much, stiffening her limbs to make him work for it.

Nice.

5 Adrian's cunnilingus-based lubrication plan has been quite successful over the years. It worked on all the girls in college, no problems, no complaints until he got married.

The Wife had a dryness problem, made worse by the fact that she didn't like foreplay at all, only fucking . . . and that not so much. Without his spit to fill the gap, he didn't know how to make her wet enough but still it never dawned on him to use personal lubrication; he thought that stuff was just for ass sex. The day the Wife told him that they should use some lubricant, he actually thought she wanted to try ass sex.

Unfortunately, having lube at hand did not magically increase the Wife's sex drive. Or maybe, by that time, it was Adrian's that had gotten desperately low. In any case, on pulling out of his marriage, lube smelled like failure.

His first lovers after the divorce only strengthened his conviction that the stuff was unnecessary. The Enthusiast and the Innocent One got wet in his mouth or hand, and the fucking worked just like before the Wife. And finally, the cherry on top: the Great One, the wettest woman he had ever known.

She got moist from a kiss. He can count on one hand the times he touched her dry snatch—must have put his hand down her pants before saying hello or something. So you can imagine that they didn't use any lube.

Then one weekend, she complained about being sore and suggested that they get some lubricant. Adrian was flabbergasted. Without communicating the unfortunate history of lube in his marriage, he cheerily agreed to go fetch some before they met again.

To prepare for the next weekend, he went to his favorite sex shop. From the hundred varieties of lube (like cereal at a grocery store), he selected one silicone and two water-soluble: unflavored and vanilla. Everyone likes vanilla, right? Not so much. It made his whole place smell like a cake shop and it made the Great One's snatch taste like flan.

Thankfully, the Great One expressed no flavor preference, so the vanilla hit the back of the drawer by noon on Saturday. The unflavored water-soluble was the next to get ash-canned. It started out OK, but at every reapplication, the stickiness increased, which accelerated the rate of reapplication . . . to the point where he was pulling out to re-lube every couple of minutes. Pretty soon, everything got so sticky that it felt like he was trying to fuck a block of taffy with a licorice stick. (Adrian has since discovered some nonglycerin, water-based lubes that don't leave any residual stickiness.)

Then the silicone. Only occasional reapplication required. Nice feeling. Neutral flavor so the Great One totally still tasted like snatch when he went back down on her. You should be warned about one drawback of silicone—it'll leave you a little slick, even after a shower. But why not leave it slippery? He'll be going back in there before you know it.

Thanks to personal lubrication, the Great One and Adrian fucked unfettered that entire weekend. Soreness? None. Overnight, lube got promoted from a squirt-bottle of frustration to the best liquid since water.

6 It took the Innocent One a long time to get around to touching Adrian's cock, but somewhere around the two-month mark, she felt the imbalance of all his finger-fucking and pussy-eating and figured that she needed to respond in kind. One night she looked

Adrian dead in the eyes, summoned her strength, and said, "You know, you can ask me to do anything . . . if there is something in particular you want me to do."

This was the most beautiful thing that anyone had ever said to Adrian Colesberry. But don't feel bad that it wasn't you. Even though you can never be the one who said it to him first, you can always be the one who's said it to him last.

That entire week, Adrian daydreamed about talking her patiently through a blowjob, but however appealing and long-awaited, her invitation also scared him to death. Teaching the Innocent One how to please him would imply a commitment to the relationship that he just didn't feel. If she started learning how to suck his cock, she'd do better week by week and after a month she'd be good and then he'd have a girlfriend.

They had talked openly about his divorce, so he could have taken the position that she'd been given fair warning and could look after her own feelings as he took what he wanted from the relationship. Plus, she said she was ready to learn. From this evidence, it seems like he was the one who couldn't handle it. Like he didn't want to let someone please him. Not completely. Not yet.

7   The way that lubrication worked its way into the lovemaking between the Great One and Adrian, he would feel a rough patch, kneel up, apply some lube to his condom, and then reenter. Looking down at the Great One during this brief reapplication process, it kind of bugged him that she was lying there with nothing to do. Not that he thought she was lazy—she'd done plenty before retiring to her back for a well-deserved rest. And not that there was time for her to learn Portuguese or anything; he was going to stick his cock back inside her within a minute. He didn't do anything about this until, one day, the Great One started casually rearranging her breast while he was re-lubing.

Before he knew what he was doing, Adrian blurted out, "Play with your nipples." He was so shocked at having said it that he wasn't really sure he'd said anything at all. But the Great One was sure about it and immediately started working her nipples between her fingers.

Accommodating reader, when Adrian asks you to do something, follow this fine example and just do it. If you ask, "What did you say?!" He'll immediately deny that he's said a word. Maybe you're not even stalling, but for the sake of accuracy, you want to double-check with him about what exactly he asked you to do. "Did you want me to touch my nipples or pinch them?" Don't double-check. Close is good enough in this situation. If you make him clarify, he's going to get so embarrassed that he won't try asking you to do anything else for a month. Your cooperation is appreciated.

From that point on, whenever he reapplied lubricant, he'd tell the Great One to do something nasty to herself, like touch her nipples or suck on her finger or stick her tongue out. Then, finally, he got his guts up and, during one re-lubing, he whispered what he really wanted her to do: "Touch yourself." His phrasing gave the both of them an out. If she didn't want to masturbate for him, she could have touched her nipples, like normal.

But once again, the Great One heard him right. She moved a hand between her legs and started masturbating. In this, as in everything, she sets a wonderful example to follow.

8   Adrian and dirty talk didn't exactly get off on the right foot, starting with the talkiest girl he ever fucked: the Talker from back in college. It was all pussy-eating and boob-handling for a few weeks, during which time she never said a word. Then the day came when she finally decided it was time for them to fuck. The second she tucked his cock inside her, she stared dead in his eyes and began rattling off an unrelenting series of questions, nodding her head insistently the whole time, to coax some response out of him, "How's that? You like the way that feels? Is that how you like it?! Uh-huh! Do you like to fuck the way I like to fuck? Tell me what you want, baby! I want to fuck you the way you want to fuck! Is that how you like it?! Tell me, baby!"

Adrian thought, "Yeah, that's how I like to fuck. But can we chat about that later? Because right now *I'm busy fucking you*!" He didn't say that, of course. In fact, he cleverly got out of saying anything at all by ramping up his pump speed and panting to give her the impression that he was way too out of breath to carry on a conversation.

The Wife made him even less comfortable with dirty talk. On the rare occasion that they stumbled into having sex, she'd say, "Fuck me!" He knew he was supposed to hear that as, "Fuck me real good!" then come back at her with something like, "Oh yeah, I'll fuck your brains out!" or "You betcha!" But since the Wife was such an incessant complainer, he didn't hear her *fuck me* as, "Fuck me real good!" Instead he heard, "Why don't you fuck me for a change, because whatever you're doing right now is *not* fucking me."

Critical reader, if a large balance of your discourse toward Adrian Colesberry consists of complaints and nags, be sure to go against the grain when dirty-talking. Use phrases that can't be interpreted as anything but praise-filled expressions of your enjoyment. Things like, "That's great!" or "I love your cock inside me." Those are hard to hear wrong.

9 Adrian's dismal opinion about dirty talk changed with the Great One. Who else? Lying around on a break one morning, she asked Adrian if he would "talk to her." He said he'd try, but immediately regretted it. He could have excused himself, "I'm sorry. I've had bad experiences with dirty talk and I don't think I can do it." But he missed his out.

As soon as they started up again, the Great One looked right into his eyes, waiting for him to say something. He fucked her until his lungs were burning and his muscles starved for oxygen, but he could only take air through his nose because he was petrified that she'd see his mouth moving and mistake a wheeze for his first attempt at dirty talk.

Her face strained in anticipation. Still, he said nothing. Another minute passed. No longer able to bear the suspense, she closed her eyes. His mind raced with possibilities: "I like my penis inside you." "You're beautiful." "I am going to fuck your brains out!" "I love your pussy." "I am so horny for you." "You have great tits."

All of it true but all of it sounding to him like lame cocktail patter at a swingers party. He was getting soft just hearing these sentences run through his head.*

---

* *Please don't let Adrian's peevish criticisms of first the Wife's and then his own dirty talk discourage you from using these exact same phrases when dirty-talking to Adrian Colesberry. "I am so horny for you" is a perfectly delightful thing to say to him while you're fucking, especially since it's the kind of thing that would counter that little voice telling him no woman really wants to have sex with him. The Wife had failed Adrian in so many ways that even her breathing pattern annoyed him. And he's equally self-critical, maybe because of all the ways that he's failed himself. But you haven't failed him at all. You can say anything.*

After Adrian rejected the common phrases, his mind returned to empty. Then it just happened. In the void, he borrowed a line from the Talker, "You like that?!" Only his pronunciation departed entirely from her approach: He didn't say it like he was demanding an answer, as she had, but with dead certainty that the Great One did like it, sounding like an Italian actor in a romantic Mafioso film, only without the accent.

"You like that?!" As he heard the words blurt out of his mouth for a second time, he felt like he had reinvented the English language. For the rest of the weekend, he didn't even bother to come up with anything else.

On the drive back home that Sunday night, he realized that he'd said "You like that?!" about a hundred times, so he called to ask the Great One to see how things had gone in the dirty-talk department.

She gave him good marks for his first outing. Apparently, dirty talk is like rock music vocals—more about attitude than quality. From that weekend forward, he talked pretty much every time they jumped in bed together. Ultimately expanding his repertoire to include dozens of phrases, including the Great One's all-time favorite: "Oh, you like it when I treat you like a dirty whore, don't you?" He could feel her get wetter when he said it.

Adrian trotted out dirty talk regularly with his girlfriends after the Great One, running aground only once: A few weeks into their relationship, the Kind One asked gingerly, "Would you mind not calling me a whore?"

10 Although it's a common enough thing for lovers to do to each other, Adrian himself wasn't aware that he personally might want to smack a woman on the ass until the very first time he saw the Innocent One. He was so shocked at the impulse that he quickly brushed it away, but no use . . . it kept coming back.

She must have sensed his desire in that direction, because one day in bed, while he was rolling her onto her stomach to change positions, he had just barely rested his hand on one of her ass cheeks when she whipped her head around to complain, "How come guys always want to smack me on the ass?!"

He hadn't smacked her ass in any way, but denial seemed hypocritical since he'd been thinking about it nonstop. So he just said, "Guys want to smack your ass because you have a stupendously great ass!" And she did. "Unless you start dating gay men," he warned her, "you should pretty much expect for guys to smack your ass."

"Well, don't," she said, not a hint of humor or coyness in her voice.

He tried to forget about it, but the more he suppressed it, the more insistent the urge became, until he decided that he would have to for-real smack her on the ass at least once—if only to get it out of his system.

Since she'd been pretty explicit in banning the smack, Adrian couldn't just up and do it. So he thought of a way to give it a context so specific that the Innocent One would be forced to admit, "Adrian's not smacking me like I clearly asked him not to. Any man would have smartly laid his hand on my ass in that situation."

His plan was to wait until she knew he was looking at her ass, like when they were lying around in bed. Then very naturally, sounding like the thought had for the first time entered his head, he'd say, "Gee, you have a great ass!" Finally, as if he wanted her to be 100 percent sure that he knew exactly which part of her body her ass was, he'd give her a sharp smack on it.

A week after she'd told him not to, he carried off his plan to smack the Innocent One's ass. They were in bed, and she was lying on her stomach. His hands were fondling her butt cheeks. He lay his foundation with the completely disarming, "Gee, you have a great ass!" Then he raised one hand a few centimeters off her ass and smacked back down on it.

She flipped over like a cat in a catfight. "I told you not to do that." Adrian had been so confident of success that he hadn't planned for failure, even though it was one of only two possible outcomes.

"But I was just . . ."

"I told you not to!" she repeated, betrayed, shocked, and on the verge of tears.

"You're right. I'm sorry. I forgot." Then he went down on her. (There aren't a lot of relationship gaffes that can't be smoothed over by offering an unadorned apology and then giving a little head. This works on Adrian Colesberry, too.)

The Innocent One didn't mention it again after he came up for air, so no harm no foul. As far as his plan to smack her ass, he figured that he hadn't laid a good enough foundation for her to understand it in the way that he'd meant it. He went off to think of a new approach before smacking her on the ass again.

11 Making out one night at her sister's boyfriend's apartment, Adrian had just pushed his fingers inside her when the Innocent One asked if he had a condom. No. He didn't have any condoms on him or even in his car.

When you start fucking Adrian Colesberry, do give the guy a little backup on the condom side. Just stick one in your purse, like in a mint tin, or in your dresser. Most likely, you'll never use it. Adrian is happy to take the responsibility for protection. It's one of the ways he shows that he cares about you—making absolutely sure you don't get knocked up or pass something to each other.

If you don't like buying condoms, that's understandable. Some people don't. Just steal a few from Adrian the first time you fuck him. He's happy to buy condoms. Tampons, too. Nothing says "I'm getting laid!" like a grocery basketful of tampons and condoms.

Of course, Adrian didn't point out to the Innocent One that she might have had a condom herself. He apologized and promised that at the next opportunity he'd stock every location—wallet, backpack, her sister's boyfriend's place. Then he resigned himself to an evening of making out and eating pussy. She persisted though, saying that there was a convenience store nearby:

Hang a right out of the apartment.

Walk down the alley between the two apartment buildings.

Take a left on the little street without the light.

Walk to the big street with the light.

Take a right, and it's two blocks dead ahead.

She swore that after the last turn he'd practically run into the register. It seemed doable. He knew he'd give in and go to the store eventually, but it was cold out so he lingered in bed for a few more seconds, enjoying the warmth.

The instant that he took a breath in preparation for sitting up, the Innocent One jumped out of bed and said, "I'll be right back." She pulled her clothes on, grabbed a few bills out of her purse, and ran out. He just lay there in total shock, staring at the closed door. She didn't want to live that night without somehow getting his cock inside her . . . and she was muling in the condoms to prove it.

The reader should steal this class move if the situation happens to repeat itself. Once he got over the shock of someone other than him doing a condom run, Adrian got undressed and tucked himself into bed . . . the least he could do was be naked and ready to go when she got back. As he pulled the covers up to his chin, he dropped off to sleep.

Her key in the door woke him up. She ripped open the box of condoms, put one on the side table, then stripped and slid between the sheets.

At the shock of her cold flesh against him, he popped an erection. The Innocent One felt it pressing into her stomach, sprung to her knees, straddled his thighs, grabbed the condom off the table, tore it open, and rolled it over his cock. It was a first for both of them: her first time touching his penis, his first time having a girl put a condom on him—mind-blowing.

Absolutely make room in your repertoire for putting a condom on Adrian Colesberry. Putting a condom on him says, "I want you to fuck me" ten times louder than your saying, "I want you to fuck me." Brilliant stuff.

After just a few strokes, the Innocent One rolled herself underneath him. She was tired from her walk and didn't want to have to do all the work. He was rested after his nap and happily took over.

So she had something after all. It wasn't cocksucking or handjobbing. The Innocent One just wanted him. That, it turned out, was a lot.

12 Adrian's habit of the wet washcloths, like most habits, didn't develop by any logical sequence of events but by a series of accidents: Right after the first time they had sex, the Kind One went into the bathroom. Before closing the door, she asked if he wanted to pee.

When you ask Adrian if he needs to pee (or if he's hungry or sleepy or in any transient physical state), he'll naturally think that you're asking if he needs to pee at the moment, not if he needs to pee again, ever. If you're planning to monopolize the bathroom for a longer-than-normal period of time, it's best to give him a more direct heads-up. Instead of "Do you need to pee?" something more like, "I'm going to be in there forever, you might want to pee."

The assertive reader may be wondering why Adrian didn't just knock on the bathroom door once he did need to and say, "Hi. I didn't need to pee when I said I didn't need to pee, but now I do need to pee." Here's the problem. The times he walked up to the door to check, he heard the Kind One contentedly humming to herself, making him think that she was conducting some important post-fuck ritual, one that he wasn't about to interrupt. So when he started dancing around because he had to pee so bad, instead of knocking, he ran back to the kitchen, stood on his toes, and started offloading his bladder into the sink.

All apologies to the clean-freak reader, but he really had to go. In his defense, urine is a nearly sterile solution and, considering his low standard of kitchen cleanliness at that time, there's little doubt that his pee-rinse left his sink better off.

He'd only just begun blasting at the stainless steel when he heard the bathroom door open. He thought about trying to squeeze it off, but that's just not possible for a guy, so he pushed it out harder instead, hoping that she'd dawdle by the door for a while like she'd dawdled in the bathroom. No such luck. As soon as she saw that he wasn't on the bed, she took a sharp left turn into the kitchen and saw him on his tiptoes hanging his tackle into the sink.

She asked him if he was jerking off. He said he wasn't. She said it was fine if he was jerking off. He said he knew it was fine but that, fine or not, he wasn't jerking off but peeing because she'd been in the bathroom for so long. The Kind One still didn't buy it. She only ended up believing him weeks later, when his masturbating in the kitchen sink after sex failed to emerge as one of his typical behaviors.

(If you do catch Adrian peeing in a sink after you fuck, instead of getting into a yes-you-are-no-I'm-not argument about whether he's jerking off, offer to hold on to his penis for him. It's fun to aim a guy's pee. Do be careful if it's your first time behind the wheel. You don't want to get pee all over the place. And no squeezing. That hurts.)

Over the time that it took for Adrian's jerking off in the sink to prove itself not to be a habit of his, the Kind One's half-hour bathroom stay became firmly established as a habit of hers. As much as he respected her privacy, he also missed her while she was gone away in there. It made him feel left out. So ultimately he felt an irresistible compulsion to somehow involve himself in her ritual.

One night, before she'd had a chance to make her move, he

popped up. "Wait a second." He started the hot water running, got her a glass of water from the kitchen, and chatted with her while the bathroom tap warmed up, then went back to the bathroom, wet a facecloth in the now-warm water, wrung it out most of the way, and proudly ran it out to the Kind One.

Thinking that it would be sensual for him to clean her snatch with the cloth, he started wiping her off. After patiently tolerating a half-minute's worth of clumsy pawing, she said, "I'll do it," took the cloth, wiped around for a bit longer, said thanks, popped up, and closed herself in the bathroom for her standard half hour—no more and certainly no less.

But Adrian is no quitter, and if you think this made him give up on shortening her bathroom time with the washcloths, you're dead wrong.

He thought, "Maybe if I bring her two cloths, one with a bit of soap on it . . ." So the next time he told her to wait, started the hot water running, got her a glass of water, chatted with her a bit, wet the cloths, wrung them out, and put a little soap on one. She cleaned off with the soapy one, wiped off with the second cloth, and closed herself in the bathroom for a half hour.

Somehow, he thought he was making progress. Since the soap hadn't affected her time in the bathroom, he concluded that, beyond a few minutes of general cleanup, the Kind One was up to something else in there. He'd been looking at this damp moist cloth thing in the wrong way. The next time . . .

He told her to wait, started the hot water running, got her a glass of water, chatted with her a bit, wet two cloths, and wrung them out. He handed her one to wipe off with. He'd palmed the second cloth and when she was done with the first, he cupped the second one against her. When she realized that he was just going to hold the warm cloth there, the Kind One relaxed and said, "Aw, that's sweet." Then she got up and closed herself in the bathroom for a half hour.

She'd called him sweet. He was on to something.

With time, he became convinced that the Kind One wasn't doing anything at all specific in the bathroom. Sex was pretty intense for her, but she couldn't have an orgasm with him. All that muscular tension she'd built up had to go somewhere and without the catastrophic relaxation of orgasm, it probably required thirty minutes to drain out of her. She wasn't engaged in some ritual, she was just hiding out in there until she'd had enough alone time to come down.

The cloths, ultimately, were nothing the Kind One needed to have. They were just Adrian's way of saying *thanks*, which was nothing she needed to hear, but something he needed to say.

Adrian's Penis: Care and Handling

A drian's penis has many manually operated functions and is designed for people who like to engage with a penis. Maybe that makes it seem like a lot of trouble, but if you think your snatch is some low-maintenance dream, you're operating under a delusion.

It might help you adopt the proper attitude if you think about Adrian's penis the same way he thinks about your ass. Stop thinking of it as *his* penis and start thinking of it as *your* penis. Not yours in a trivial capitalist sense, like it's property, but more like it's a field of beans that a farmer has planted right behind her house. She cares for the field all year long. She knows when to feed and water it, when to work the field, and when to let it rest. In the following, find instructions on how to feed, water, work, and rest Adrian's penis.

Adrian's Shy Erection

Sexually demanding reader, please don't envision a constantly floppy Adrian Colesberry daily inventing new excuses for his defective arousal mechanism. Aside from occasionally being knocked out by drink, his cock has proven reliable over the years with two exceptions: in the getting-to-know-you part of the relationship and again when the relationship is going badly.[1]

A typical first time with Adrian Colesberry plays out like a physical comedy routine where every time the thirsty heroine bends down to the water fountain, the stream retreats to a dribble. He'll go down on you until he gets his erection, but he'll lose it as soon as he reaches for the condom. If you're kind enough, you'll get him hard again in your hand or mouth, but right when he tears open the condom, he'll go all floppy again.

You may be perfectly willing to keep sucking his cock, and while your generosity will be more than welcome, it'll just make Adrian feel weird after a bit to be in your mouth without getting hard enough fast enough.

Tip: *When Adrian is having his first-time erection problems, there is such a thing as paying too much attention to his cock.*

The generous reader might have been looking forward to sucking Adrian's flaccid penis to erection. But not knowing how to judge if he's getting "hard enough, fast enough," how will you know when to abandon your project of making him hard in your mouth? You needn't be concerned about the timing. Adrian will remove his cock from your mouth if he's getting self-conscious, and switch you to another activity. Another activity means, of course, more pussy-eating. As long as his shy erection is in town, he'll eat your pussy until his tongue cramps up—like way toward the back and even in his neck, where all the tongue muscles are attached.

The sensitive reader may be overly worried about what exactly to do when Adrian's shy erection shows up. Don't be. You can do anything that makes you feel like you're helping out, because Adrian's erection problems will go away on your second or third time regardless of what you do.[2]

Your cure for Adrian's shy erection is like your mom's cure for a cold. A cold cures itself, but your mom wants to feel like she's doing something to take care of you, so she makes you soup or gives you a pill and when you get better, she feels like she had a part in it. In the same way, do whatever you like to help fix Adrian's shy erection and when a few days later he's fucking your brains out, you'll feel like you have somehow helped make that happen. Throw a penny into a fire, light incense in an abalone shell, masturbate for him, read him French poetry. It'll all work.

And remember, while you wait for his penis to come online, someone who combines the desperate enthusiasm of a sixteen-year-old boy with the know-how of a grown man will be munching on your box for hours. Assuming you enjoy cunnilingus, everything will work out just fine.

Adrian's Reluctant Orgasm

It takes a long time for Adrian to cum with a woman; always has. It can't be a physical thing, because he cums easily when he's masturbating. But it will be several weeks or months into your relationship before he has an orgasm with you. The experienced reader may be hearing this with a shake of the head: "Adrian won't last two minutes with me. There's this thing I do with my tongue/finger/vagina . . ." Perhaps, but read on.

Perfection

Best that can be figured, Adrian's overactive cum suppression mechanism got Frankensteined together when the standard propaganda about how a man has to last forever in the sack grafted itself onto his trained-from-the-womb perfectionism.

Whenever he did anything, like take a shit or recite a multiplication table or bring home a piece of child-art made from paste and pinto beans, his mother would say, "Little Adrian, you're just perfect." He knew it wasn't true, but in an effort not to disappoint the kindly woman who'd brought him into this world, he did his best to keep up the front by behaving the way he thought a perfect person would behave.

It's Baby Adrian who puts the brakes on when he gets close to orgasm, "What are you doing, Adrian? We're not supposed to cum."

Adrian tries to explain, "It's only at first that we're not supposed to."

"How are we going to last forever if you cum?"

"It's not literally 'forever.'"

"I've heard it's 'forever.'"

"She already came. That's why we went down on her for so long. Now we can go ahead."

"That's not how I understood it."

Then Adrian gets all mad, like, "That's because you're what? Six?! You don't understand anything. Just let me cum!" But by that time the window of opportunity has closed again.

It's not that he doesn't get close. He can cum easily in the first thirty seconds. But he always holds back because he doesn't want to prematurely ejaculate. That would make him a premature ejaculator. Plus, he doesn't want to stop having sex so soon after starting. On taking the first bite of his favorite meal, his next thought after "That's delicious!" is not "Gee, I hope this experience ends immediately."

A ways after that first one, a second window of opportunity arrives, but by the time he recognizes it, an automatic part of his brain has already taken over and stifled his orgasm again (see sidebar on page 84). And so it goes with the third window and the fourth.[3]

The cynical reader might suspect that this up-to-now objective account of how to make love to Adrian Colesberry has been corrupted by a crass attempt to promote Adrian Colesberry's sexual athleticism, that this complaint about his not being able to cum is obviously meant to imply that his lovemaking will be lengthy, and that the next chapter will contain an equally transparent moan about the inconvenient girthiness of his cock. Not at all!

Adrian holds no delusions about a woman wanting a man to last forever. In his experience, they resoundingly haven't. It's great for those first few times when you just can't get enough of each other, but after that, if you are anything like every woman he's ever been with, you'll be over it. Following the zero, one, or several orgasms you want to have, Adrian's erection turns from a fun new toy into a party guest who won't leave at the end of the evening. "Oh, that's still there. Do I have to do something about it?"

The answer is an emphatic no. You don't have to do anything about it. Adrian enjoys fucking more than cumming. If he just wants to cum, he won't bother fucking you in the first place; he'll jerk off. So just call *time* when you're done and he's all good.

In Adrian's experience, the trickiest part of his not cumming will be managing your frustration. If you're accustomed to having the power to bring off a man with your hand, mouth, or vagina, the discovery that you don't have your finger on the trigger of Adrian Colesberry might not make you happy.[4]

Faking It

In most every relationship in his life, Adrian, a reasonably faithful condom user, could have faked an orgasm while fucking just to make a lady smile. But he never has and never will. There's something about the ethics of that small-seeming lie that he finds deeply disrespectful. If you're in a relationship with Adrian, there must be a tacit agreement between the two of you never to lie about that issue.

If you have lied already, that's not the end or anything. Just tell him. He will be hurt, but he'll get over it and when he does, the two of you can return to square one and figure out together how you like to get fucked.

The sensitive reader may perceive a profound ungenerousness or distancing mechanism in Adrian's not achieving the ultimate sexual pleasure. You may hear his never cumming as "I don't really need you." Please do not indulge this train of thought. If Adrian is fucking you, he needs you.

Adrian's Ejaculation

Ultimately, Adrian will start having orgasms with you. The following chart presents how these will be distributed, based on a review of the historical data.

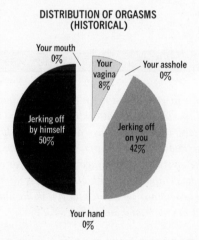

DISTRIBUTION OF ORGASMS
(HISTORICAL)

Your mouth
0%

Your vagina
8%

Your asshole
0%

Jerking off by himself
50%

Jerking off on you
42%

Your hand
0%

First, you'll have noticed the null sets associated with Adrian cumming in your mouth, asshole, or hand. The fact that he never has in the past doesn't mean it won't happen in the future, but judging from historical data it's nothing you need to plan for.

Second, note that even in a relationship Adrian will be working out around half his orgasms on his own. This isn't because he likes himself more than he likes you. It's because he wants his sex drive to be a blessing for you, not a burden, so he will adjust the number of orgasms he has with you to a quantity that your own sex drive will happily accommodate.

Third, even when Adrian does have orgasms with you, 84 percent of them will result from him jerking off on you.[5] Knowing this, it's important to think about what parts of your body you'd like Adrian to jerk off on. In order of preference he'd pick your mouth, your ass, your tits, then your stomach. He'll ask before he jerks off on anything, but he'll more or less assume that it's OK for him to jerk off on your stomach or on your ass. He absolutely will not move beyond that without more explicit discussion. But if you're all good with his jerking off in your mouth or on your tits, don't let him spend months splitting time between your stomach and your ass. Throw the man an upgrade. He'll really appreciate it.

Cum in Your Eye?

Getting cum in your eye stings a bit. No wonder. There are thousands of sperm in there, attacking your cornea like it's the outer membrane of an ovum. Eye drops won't help, but don't worry, Adrian knows something that will. It's a rinse that his father used whenever Baby Adrian got something or other in his eyes. Adrian has employed it with great success on his lovers in the past, and he will mix up a batch for you in the unlikely event that he misses the mark and jacks off in your eye.

PAPA COLESBERRY'S CUM-TESTED SALINE EYE WASH
In a clean mug, dissolve a couple of tablespoons pure sea salt in warm water. Pour portions of the saline into a standard shot glass. Press the rim of the glass as close as you can get against your eye. Tilt your head back and blink. After repeated irrigation, the stinging will stop and your eye will feel as good as new. His father sure knew a lot about things.

Thanks, Papa Colesberry.

Know that once you let him jerk off in your mouth/face, he'll assume that you don't want cum in your eyes or ear holes and he will never off-load everything in your mouth—he's not trying to make a porn movie. When cumming in your mouth, he'll start there then quickly move to the pillow or your tits. He's got a lot of practice with follow-up re-aiming, so you'll just have a couple of drops to spit out. Above all, don't start telling him where to aim when he's in the middle of things. Adrian has a hard time cumming in the best of circumstances. If you're calling out stuff like "Not in my navel!" he doesn't have a chance.

To avoid all of these difficulties, mark on the drawing below those spots where you'd be happy for Adrian to jerk off on.

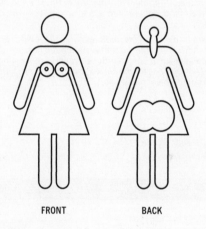

FRONT   BACK

Your Orgasms Together

To help you to think about your orgasms with Adrian Colesberry, the women in his experience have been arranged into four groups by style: the auto-orgasmic, the non-orgasmic, the Adrian-orgasmic and finally, the combination Adrian- and auto-orgasmic.[6] As you try to imagine which category you'll fit into, don't think about these groupings as a progression of virtue or steps in a development. Each type is a variation. Regardless of your bodily habits or beliefs, each type may not need to progress or change in any way. Each category has delivered essential lessons in lovemaking, but most important, each has proven that its kind is fully capable of pleasing and being pleased by Adrian Colesberry.

KEY TO AROUSAL GRAPHS:

⌇	Woman's arousal level
∿	Adrian's arousal level
Y-axis	Arousal scale, units unassigned (Each graph would of course require two Y-axes, one representing Adrian's arousal and one representing the woman's. To obtain the current graphs, the scales were normalized then superimposed such that the orgasm thresholds were perfectly overlapping.)
X-axis	Time scale (duration of lovemaking or time period during which Adrian and the woman both achieved orgasm, whichever was longer)
	Orgasm threshold. This midline marks the level of arousal above which Adrian and the woman experienced orgasm. The time a particular arousal line spends above this orgasm line does not represent the length of a climax, but the period during which a climax could be achieved.

The auto-orgasmic woman

Lesson #1.

Adrian cannot make you have an orgasm, but he can help.

Twenty-seven percent of the women in Adrian's past have reached orgasm only ever by masturbating. In all these cases, Adrian did find a way to assist them.

Lesson #2.

Ladies first.

Not only is Adrian fully indoctrinated in the commonplace virtue of ensuring a woman has had her orgasm before taking his own, he leans toward not involving his penis in activities at all until a woman has cum. He understands that this isn't always the way a woman wants things to go down and under no circumstances will he make your orgasm some hurdle you have to jump over before you get to play with his cock; you can play with his cock whenever you like. His extreme interpretation of the Ladies First rule does, however, explain some of his behavior, his near religious devotion to eating pussy for one.

AUTO-ORGASMIC, EXHIBIT A[7]

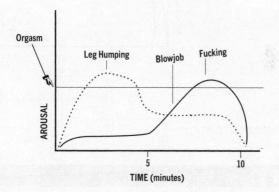

AUTO-ORGASMIC, EXHIBIT B[8]

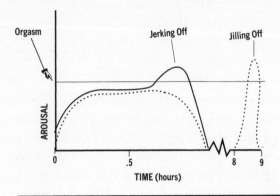

AUTO-ORGASMIC, EXHIBIT C[9]

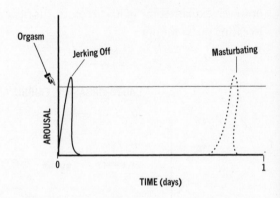

The non-orgasmic woman

Lesson #3.

If a woman can't have an orgasm while masturbating or doesn't masturbate at all, Adrian's help isn't going to be all that helpful.

Adrian's penis, mouth, and fingers aren't magical (sorry). If you haven't figured out how to give yourself an orgasm on your own, there's not much chance that he's going to come riding in with the solution. But sex is very pleasant without an orgasm; just ask Adrian Colesberry, who hasn't cum in the majority of his own sexual encounters.

It's not that he'll give up after hearing the news that it hasn't happened for you. If you want to try, Adrian will bar no effort to help you get off however many times and in whatever way you want. But at the same time, Adrian won't hang his manhood on the number, strength, or screaminess of your orgasms, and he's not going to do anything that makes you feel lesser-than by turning your orgasm, or lack of one, into a watched pot.

The way he sees it, once everyone's clothes come off, it's all a good time. Fucking toward a goal, even if that goal is something pretty nice like an orgasm, allows the concept of failure to enter into an arena where it just doesn't belong. Adrian doesn't enjoy fucking under pressure to cum and won't put you through that either.

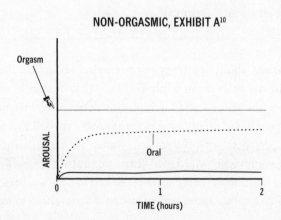

NON-ORGASMIC, EXHIBIT A[10]

NON-ORGASMIC, EXHIBIT B[11]

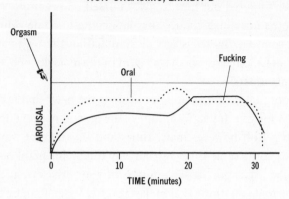

The Adrian-orgasmic woman

Lesson #4.

It's not all about the clitoris.

Having learned about sex from pornographic epistolary literature, Adrian was miseducated into thinking that he should more or less locate the clitoris and latch on to it like a dog on a bone until the woman had an orgasm. He profoundly revised this idea after his experiences with the several women whose orgasms relied on his competent help. Upon learning that they didn't just want him to latch on to their clitorises, he had to broaden his view of women's erogenous zones before he could assist them to satisfactory climaxes.

ADRIAN-ORGASMIC, EXHIBIT A[12]

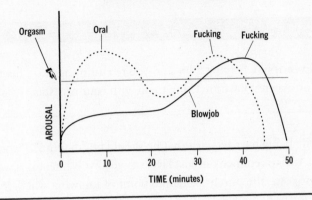

ADRIAN-ORGASMIC, EXHIBIT B[13]

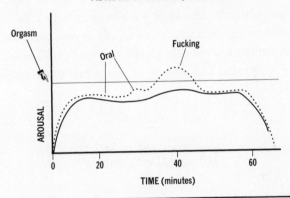

ADRIAN-ORGASMIC, EXHIBIT C[14]

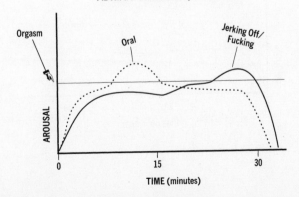

Lesson #5.

Even if he's helping a lot and you're cumming a lot, his help may or may not have anything to do with your orgasms.

Despite being over the idea that he should be "making" a woman cum, Adrian retained one last layer of ego-involvement in a woman's orgasm: the purely academic point of knowing whether she was cumming by herself or due to anything he was doing. After several experiences with women who were as all over themselves as he was, Adrian let this layer wash away as well. Your inviting Adrian to participate in whatever capacity in your orgasmic experience is plenty good enough. Maybe you don't even know exactly how it's happening and as long as you're cumming why would anyone care?

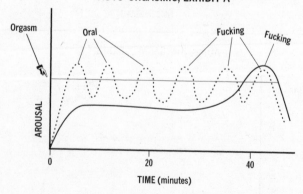

COMBINATION ADRIAN-ASSISTED AUTO-ORGASMIC, EXHIBIT A[15]

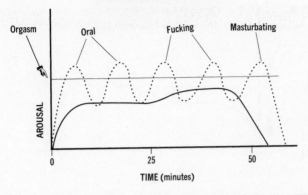

COMBINATION ADRIAN-ASSISTED AUTO-ORGASMIC, EXHIBIT B[16]

Orgasm

Oral   Fucking   Masturbating

AROUSAL

0   25   50

TIME (minutes)

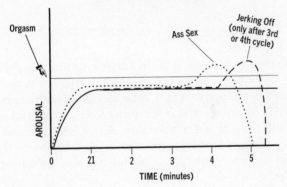

COMBINATION ADRIAN-ASSISTED AUTO-ORGASMIC, EXHIBIT C[17]

Orgasm

Ass Sex   Jerking Off (only after 3rd or 4th cycle)

AROUSAL

0   21   2   3   4   5

TIME (minutes)

You

The graph on the next page has one orgasm line, representing Adrian's typical cycle. Draw in your own pattern. If your line rises above the orgasm line, indicate what, if anything, Adrian can do to help you have that orgasm. Also put units on the time scale, (minutes or hours) and numbers on the hash marks to indicate how long you'd like to fuck.

YOU

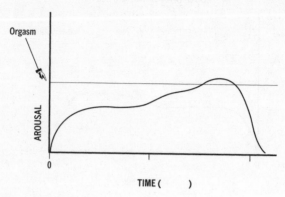

CHAPTER 5 NOTES

1   There have been two times in Adrian's life when his shy erection has not been a temporary, up-front problem: with the Wife and once before that with the Deliberate One. We can breeze over the Wife by assuming that you won't force Adrian exclusively into the roles of father, caretaker, doctor, and provider, not leaving any part for his penis to play because Adrian the father-caretaker-doctor-provider will not fuck his child-invalid-patient-ward.

The Deliberate One offers a far more instructive example of how Adrian's erection can be driven into hibernation. She lived at the women's dorm where Adrian was a waiter in college. He became part of her drinking circle and ended up with a little bit of a crush on her, which grew into a lot a bit of a crush once he learned that her main goal in college, aside from graduating of course, was to fuck at least one person other than her high-school boyfriend who was the man she'd given her virginity to and the man she planned to marry after college. A noble cause. Needless to say, Adrian wanted to sign up.

Tip: *Historically speaking, people have underexploited the ability to help themselves reach their potential by fucking Adrian Colesberry. If you have any life goals that he can help along in this way, please let him know.*

Adrian soon learned from another girl in their circle that the Deliberate One had chosen him to do the fucking. So with no fear of rejection, he asked her out. For their first few dates, they just necked in his car, but eventually, he got her over to his place and before the evening was done, she let him take her pants off.

He went down on her for a long time using everything he'd learned between the Loved One's legs. When he came up for air, she lay back in anticipation of his entry. And then was when he lost his erection. At that moment, he could have said truthfully, for the first and the last time, "I swear, this has never happened to me before." He felt sure that the problem would pass, but it didn't. Weeks went by and they were only ever about boob handling and eating pussy.

Unless your fantasy affair with Adrian Colesberry involves him going down on you and a lot of making out, he's apparently not the greatest guy to fuck around with on your boyfriend or husband. On the other hand, he's older now, of course, and the Deliberate One is not you, unless it is you. So maybe Adrian and, more important, Adrian's penis, would be thrilled to be one half of the adulterous affair you'd like to have behind the back of your lucky someone. Just don't put a down payment on a condo/love nest until you test-drive his cock for a bit.

Knowing how much she wanted to fuck someone else, Adrian felt really guilty about not being able to get it up for her. It was like a terminal cancer patient had asked him to give her a fuck before dying, but he couldn't because of his ridiculous, uncooperative erection. Then it dawned on him that maybe she could do something to make it more cooperative. In his first-ever attempt at asking anyone to do him a favor in bed, he asked if she had ever considered sucking his cock. She had, so that was good, but she said she only did that for her boyfriend. Afterward, he no longer felt guilty about not being able to fuck her.

Depending on your perspective, Adrian's impotence in this

case was triggered either by a respectful objection to the Deliberate One's infidelity or by her lack of physical attention. The monogamous, blowjob-averse reader should choose to believe that Adrian's sense of rectitude kept his penis flaccid; the adulterous reader should choose to believe that he's one enthusiastic blowjob away from getting hard enough to fuck the pope's girlfriend.

2   Adrian has experienced a wide range of reactions to his shy erections. Despite her name or maybe because of it, the Great One did make the beautiful mistake of sucking his cock for an uncomfortably long time in an attempt to get it up. His problems lasted a particularly short time with the Innocent One, who never once touched it. No credit to her though; she barely touched his penis at all, shy or otherwise. The Last One more deliberately ignored the early erection difficulties, to the extent that when he mentioned it, she didn't even speak, like she hadn't heard him. Good move.

The Talker, from back in college, and the Expert had the most hysterical responses to his shy erection. The Talker imagined that his enthusiasm was flagging due to a lack of kink and flipped into every conceivable sexual position to inspire him. Eighteen years later, the Expert also chose to up the kink: after an abortive bout of doggie-style, she did an acrobatic maneuver where she ended up with her legs wrapped around his neck, putting them into a standing 69 where she deep-throated him. That worked for a bit, but when she came up for air, Adrian still didn't have enough to pull a condom over.

At this point, she spun into a total panic. Her alarm grew and grew until she blurted out, "I'm going to ask my mom for one of Dad's pills." Apparently, her father took an erection pill to get hard.

Adrian started to tell her for the one-millionth time that his penis would work OK soon enough, but she looked so utterly lost at having failed to generate a hard cock in the way that she was used to. So he changed his mind and said, "Fantastic. Definitely ask your mother."

He felt quite generous about his assent. Not only did it make the Expert happy but it'd give Dad a thrill to hear that some young stud, relatively speaking, needed a bit of the same chemical assistance that he needed himself. Mainly though, he wanted to hear the Expert report on the conversation where she asked her mother for one of her husband's pills. "Thanks for the hard-on pills, Mom. Keep 'em coming, and this guy you've never met can pork your daughter." Words every girl's mother dreams of hearing.

Moving from the absurd to the sublime, the prizewinning responses to Adrian's early loss of erection belong to the Enthusiast and the Kind One: When Adrian fell to half mast, the Enthusiast would lie down beside him, cup his balls in one hand and, with her other hand, she'd masturbate herself. To break down why this is so brilliant, grabbing his balls maintained contact with his naughty bits, but not a part that needs to do anything, so he couldn't interpret her touch as a demand of any kind. And the masturbation communicated that she hadn't taken their forced break as a failure. She was going to be sexually satisfied whether he could fuck her or not. That made him feel a lot better.

The Kind One pulled a maneuver of even greater genius, if you can imagine it. At his first failure, she jumped off the bed, grabbed some lotion from the bedside table, and gave him a foot massage. Saying without saying, "I'm going to love you whether your penis is on board or not." Not only was this the kindest maneuver, but it got the quickest result. He was fucking her within five minutes.

3 The only person to break Adrian's reluctant orgasm was the First One. It remains controversial what exactly caused his orgasm to flip from reluctant to nearly immediate. All the evidence for all points of view will be presented here in a balanced way so that you can make up your own mind.

Once she decided that they were an item, Adrian became the beneficiary of the First One's girlfriend ethics:

- *The primary rule:* Any time she found Adrian with a hard-on, it was her job to make it go away.
- *The secondary rule:* She was responsible for harvesting all his semen.

The lawyerly reader might object that the secondary rule is simply a corollary of the primary. But although the primary rule provides the foundation for the second, it is not a sufficient condition. The primary rule only required that she solved the erections that she found. The secondary rule required her to be there to find all his erections, something she did with near perfect fidelity. Often at great inconvenience to herself, she would spend every night with

Adrian. He thought at first that she was doing all this on account of a deep affection but really it was an ethical imperative, as follows:

The First One is Adrian's girlfriend iff the First One harvests all Adrian's Semen.
The First One harvests all Adrian's Semen iff the First One sleeps over every night.
∴
The First One sleeps over every night.

QED

[Where iff = if and only if, in other words the singular sufficient condition(s).]

At night, she'd get there just before he went to bed and they'd fuck until he came. Then they'd sleep until his second erection woke up one of them at around three in the morning, then they'd fuck again. Then she'd take care of his morning erection, of course, after which she'd promptly leave for work.

This pattern wasn't immediately established. His reluctant orgasm heroically persisted for several weeks before he came for the first time, but once she'd gotten her foot in the door, she had him cumming progressively quicker. Within two weeks, he'd stopped masturbating altogether because she was keeping up with his testicles' production capacity. Adrian, as you can imagine, felt a bit confused and unmanned by the arrangement. He was hardly lasting forever as he knew he should be. But the First One's positive attitude, driven by her high level of girlfriend accomplishment as defined by her own ethics, convinced him that everything was OK.

Besides, she would already have had an orgasm by the time she tucked his cock inside her since she came beforehand by humping his thigh, so Adrian ultimately was able to cast a positive light on lasting barely three minutes: He hadn't begun to prematurely ejaculate. *Not at all!* What he'd done was custom-develop a hyperefficient style of lovemaking. Fucking was pointless for her since she wouldn't have another orgasm with him inside her. So in his genius, he'd cut it down to a bare minimum.

The first theory to explain his unusual behavior is called the Masturbation Substitution Theory. It holds that if you (or anyone) were to arrange your life such that you're ready and willing to fuck at least as frequently as Adrian would masturbate, he'd ultimately make the switch and fuck you in place of masturbating, which would automatically endow your lovemaking with the ejaculatory efficiency of his masturbation.

This conventional explanation faces a challenge from the Mononucleosis Hypothesis. Some have correctly pointed out that, halfway through the relationship, Adrian contracted mononucleosis from the First One. Theory holds that the catastrophic impact on his immune system had the side effect of making him a premature ejaculator.

The curious reader, if annoyed at how Adrian rarely cums, could stage an experiment, first try harvesting all his semen and then infect him with a virus—nothing too serious, please—and see which technique makes him ejaculate faster.

4   After he'd gone to all that trouble using the 69 to finesse the Loved One into giving him head, Adrian found her fellatio disappointingly tepid. One night, lying there with his cock in her barely animated mouth, everything suddenly became crystal clear to him: Her old boyfriend had shot off in her mouth without warning and she thought that was going to happen with Adrian, too, bringing their fun to an end. He thought, "Good news! I can clear up this misunderstanding in a jiffy!"

Raising his head off the mattress, he happily announced, "You know there's no way I'm ever going to cum in your mouth, so you don't have to worry about that at all!" Now he figured she could relax and enjoy sucking his cock as much as he enjoyed eating her pussy, but instead of the reassurance he had intended, she took his statement as a mortal insult against her cocksucking skills. She heard "You give head so lousy that you could stay down there till next Tuesday and I'd never have it off."

In response to his unintended challenge, the Loved One pushed her cocksucking to heights of hair-raising intensity. She encouraged him to ejaculate in her mouth, even before he'd fucked her. "I've got a washcloth right here to spit out in!" After dishing out several servings of the best blowjob that came out of her kitchen, she got positively panicky about getting him off. To give her some hope to hang on to, he abandoned the position that busting his nut during head would be impossible and took to promising that he was seriously getting very close to getting off.

A few weeks into the Loved One's blowjob-ejaculation project,

Adrian finally came while fucking her. He was so surprised that he completely forgot what they'd been going through and reverted to being worried that he'd cum too soon. "Were you done?!" She gave him a look like, "Yeah, I was done two months ago."

5 Adrian never had an orgasm with the Enthusiast or with the Innocent One. It may surprise you to learn that he never came with the Great One either, but it was with her that he began his efforts to jerk off on someone. The first person to suggest that Adrian jerk off on the Great One was, oddly enough, not the Great One but his psychotherapist. She didn't exactly say he should do it *on* the Great One. She merely pointed out, quite logically, that since he could cum easily while masturbating, he should be able to masturbate with someone else in the room.

At first take, the idea really turned him off. This seems enormously two-faced, seeing how much he enjoyed watching the Great One masturbate, but to the exact extent that female masturbation seems beautiful to him, male masturbation seems repellant. On those occasions when he catches himself in a mirror, he sees a monkey in a tree . . . just jerking off until it's time to fling a turd at someone.

The Saturday after his therapist had made her suggestion, he collapsed exhausted beside the Great One, ready for the long break from fucking that they called early evening, when she suggested, "Why don't you jerk off on me?" Spooky! Were she and his therapist calling each other to plot his progress? Even though he'd been set up to accept the idea, he declined right off the bat, saying he was too self-conscious to go through with it.

Then two Sundays later, the going got rough so he pulled out and knelt between her parted legs to reapply some lubricant. While he coated the condom, she closed her eyes and started fingering herself. Mesmerized by her masturbation, a few minutes passed before he realized that he was either doing the most thorough lubricant reapplication of all time or he was jerking himself off through the condom.

Once he became aware of it, he pulled his hand away, but the instant he did the Great One ordered, "Don't stop!" That's when he noticed her eyes were not totally shut. She had closed them like louvers, blocking out from her visual field everything that wasn't Adrian's hand stroking his cock.

She told him to take the condom off, so he did and then continued jerking off, this time with the purpose of cumming on her stomach. He got close, but he couldn't.

The next day, she was giving him head when it dawned on Adrian that he might be able to cum by half letting her suck him off and half jerking off on her. He'd seen it dozens of times in porn—guys cumming on a girl's face—and porn girls couldn't get enough of the stuff. They acted like cum was the elixir of youth.

Alarmed reader, Adrian knows that porn girls are pretending and that he can't expect a real girl to behave like that. But he also knew that the Great One would honestly tell him what she would or would not want him to do. So, he asked her if he could jerk off on her face. The Great One, living up to her name, gave him the green light as long as he didn't cum in her hair.

With the hair prohibition established, the Great One gave him head for a while. Then he pulled out and jerked off toward her open mouth. Then he gave it back to her so she could suck his cock again. They swapped off like that for a while. The entire time, he used his free hand to keep her hair swept behind her. That's right. Adrian listens.

In case you're worried that this is heading toward a spit/swallow thing, it isn't. Adrian doesn't care about that. The way he figures it, once his semen travels outside of his body, it's not his decision what to do with it any longer. Besides, the Great One had told him up front that she didn't swallow. At the same time, getting it in her mouth didn't worry him because she'd told him that his cum tasted good—a judgment she'd made from his pre-cum. She didn't mean that he tasted like honey or Turkish delight. She was just saying that, considering all the men who had cum in her mouth, his cum had a better than average flavor. That was nice to hear.

Tip: *Adrian certainly isn't begging for compliments on the taste of his cum. But if it dawns on you to say a little something, do. Long before you get around to that, he'll have said how he finds your juice box a saucy delight, so it'll only be returning the favor.*

Prior to being clued in, Adrian had no idea how his cum might rank in a taste test. He'd never tasted another man's, so he didn't have anything to compare with. He had of course sampled his own brand, which he found chalky and a bit bitter, but not gross.

When he shared his self-evaluation with the Great One, she reassured him that all cum had a chalky base but that the bitterness level, aroma, backbone, and aftertaste varied depending on diet and health. She said, "If your cum is sour, eating parsley will make it taste better." The reader with a refined palate might encourage Adrian to eat parsley before he starts cumming in your mouth.* Maybe make a point of going on dates to Middle Eastern restaurants and ordering large bowls of tabbouleh to share.

Adrian never managed to cum on the Great One that day, and they broke up before he could relax enough to pull it off. But one night with the Kind One, he got too tired to fuck any longer and ended up standing at the side of the bed, finger-fucking her while she gave him head. Then he asked if he could jerk off in her mouth. He hadn't tried this with the Kind One yet.

A few minutes later, he was pointing at her open mouth when it started. Never having jerked off on anyone in his life, he found himself without an aiming strategy. The first bit got in her mouth, which was quite the point really, but she flinched in a reflexive reaction so he moved his penis up (from the frying pan into the fire), and came in her hair and a bit in her eye (see sidebar on page 88), then he pointed groundward and emptied the rest right onto the pillow, where he should have re-aimed in the first place.

6 Seeing as men are notorious at overpredicting women's orgasms, the skeptical reader might wonder how exactly Adrian determined their occurrence in his ladies. Good question. In many cases, women have been kind enough to give him verbal clues like "I'm cumming," or "Don't touch me there anymore, I just came," or "I'm finished, do you want to jerk off now?" In addition, Adrian has long been aware that a woman's orgasm is accompanied by vaginal contractions set at 0.8-second intervals. These are quite easy to detect, especially when his face is right up inside your hole

---

* *The Great One warned him that if he started smoking, even the parsley thing wouldn't help. Apparently, a smoker's cum tastes super-gross regardless. This fascinating piece of trivia makes one think that the antismoking folks are going about their business in the wrong way.*

and, while not impossible to fake, a woman would have to know this obscure fact and incorporate some appropriately spaced voluntary contractions into her raging-orgasm act to get it by Adrian Colesberry.

7 THE FIRST ONE

Adrian Colesberry's first auto-orgasmic woman was his first woman, period. After making out for a while, the First One would flip on top of him and hump his leg for five minutes until she got off. After and only after she'd secured her own orgasm would she start involving his penis in any activities. Experience had taught her to get hers before a man's ejaculation had dampened his enthusiasm for the project.

Her procedure was great by Adrian since it really took the pressure off—all he had to do for her to cum was just lie there. Good thing, too, because with the First One humping away on top of him, lying there was all he could do. She was a big girl—not meaning grown-up, but meaning fat. With her on top of him, he could move his arms and his eyes and not much more. He felt like an insect pinned to a display board, except instead of a pin it was like a squishy anvil.

Always the first to clear dishes at a party, Adrian cheerily offered up one evening, "Anything I can do to help out?" She must have been waiting for him to ask because she immediately shot back, "You can pinch my nipples."

Her nipples were smashed against his chest, but she didn't lift up to give him access. Not wanting to interrupt her leg humping a second time, Adrian took it upon himself to solve the problem of how to get at them. He twisted his torso one way then another until his hands were pressed between their two chests like collected wildflowers. Now reduced to moving only his eyes, he tweaked and pinched and rolled her hard, cough-drop-shaped nipples between each forefinger and thumb. In subsequent outings, he asked some questions to make sure he was doing it the way she liked—not too hard, not too soft. He's helpful.

8 THE KIND ONE

Adrian had been going out with the Kind One for a few months before he asked if there was anything he could do to help her have an orgasm. She said there was nothing and assured him that she was having a very good time. Then one morning, about an hour after she'd left him, the Kind One called from her home to ask, "What happened last night?" He reminded her of a few things they'd done, then she asked a follow-up question then another and another until he realized that she wasn't being forgetful and wanting to be reminded; they were having phone sex. She'd never had an orgasm in his bed, but by the time they hung up, she'd had two. So that's what she did. She drove home afterward and masturbated. When he later asked her how, she said that she humped a pillow or a champagne bottle wrapped in a towel. In this case, Adrian had helped by providing the fucking in the first place and then by helping her recollect her memories of it while she got herself off.

9 THE WIFE

Adrian generally masturbated in the morning before he went to work while the Wife was asleep. She masturbated at night while he was asleep by humping the couch arm.[*] Their couch didn't have rectangular arms with edges but puffy, upholstered arms that were quite well suited for humping away on. You may wonder how Adrian was helping in this situation, being that he was asleep in the next room: Adrian had paid for the couch.

10 THE DELIBERATE ONE

The Deliberate One was well-endowed labia-wise. When Adrian tongue-fucked her, it was like he was wearing an oxygen mask . . . made of snatch. There was so much real estate to cover that he didn't know what to do at first. Her clitoris was way too sensitive to be touched, so he roamed around her labia and then every once in a while put on the oxygen mask and buried his face in her hole.

---

* *Some readers might be surprised at how frequently Adrian has encountered women who masturbate by humping. It's hard to know whether this frequency is surprising or not, as reliable statistics about women's masturbation styles are difficult to come by in the general population. Fortunately, numbers are easy to come by with the eleven women experienced by Adrian Colesberry: Only one failed to report her masturbation style (9 percent), one reported not masturbating at all (9 percent), six masturbated with fingers and/or a vibrator (55 percent), and three masturbated by humping or grinding against something like a pillow or a couch arm or Adrian Colesberry himself (27 percent). If you fall into that last category, you'll be happy to know that Adrian has several body parts that have been humped to good effect: his erection, his foot, his thigh, his face (go easy), and his hand laid palm-down on a mattress. Take your pick of these, or appropriate some other part for your purposes.*

Halfway through his third trip between her legs, he asked if he was giving her orgasms. At the time, it seemed like a stupid question because she was soaking wet before he even got down there and she had made a Thanksgiving-turkey-platter-sized wet spot on the bed by the time he finished. He was half-convinced that the Deliberate One came on the car ride over to his place and his cunnilingus was just icing on top, so you can imagine his shock when she told him that she'd never had an orgasm . . . in her life . . . not with her one-and-only boyfriend, not even masturbating, never.

Once she mentioned it though, he paid closer attention and noticed that her vagina didn't go through the spasmodic contractions he'd become used to. Figuring that her previous boyfriend was just a lousy lover, he took her anorgasmia as a personal challenge and redoubled his efforts to pleasure her gigantic snatch.

Jump forward to four orgasm-free months later when his attitude toward her boyfriend had changed to "That man's a champ. He did his best."

11 THE INNOCENT ONE

At first, the orgasmic pattern of the Innocent One seemed easy to detect. After ten minutes or so of the upside-down *V* thing that the Loved One had taught him and his elsewise roaming around, the muscles in her legs would tighten, she'd push up her hips, start shaking, then abruptly, she'd drag his face up out of her box and have him fuck her. She might or might not have cum again while fucking; he couldn't tell and didn't press for details, thinking it might make her self-conscious.

She seemed to be enjoying the head so much already that he didn't even rush to ask the critical question about how she masturbated: pillow-humping or finger work/vibrator and, when he finally did get around to asking her, he was more or less just looking to get a hard-on by having the Innocent One describe how she got herself off. So imagine his shock when, in response to his question, she whispered, "I don't." Who doesn't masturbate?!

Masturbation relieves stress and teaches you how to please yourself, giving you valuable tips that you can pass on to Adrian Colesberry. At the same time, he also realizes that it's not for everyone. So you certainly don't have to masturbate, just if you do, describe it to him in detail.

On his next trip between her legs, Adrian paid extra-close

attention to the exact mechanics of what he had previously thought to be her orgasm. Yes, her legs tensed up, and yes, she did start to grind into his face, and yes, her whole body started shaking, but her snatch never went through that spasmodic tension and relaxation that he had experienced with the orgasms of other women.

He knew that different women climaxed in different ways and that the Innocent One's orgasm might happen without all that, but in light of the fact that she had never made herself cum by masturbating, her reactions were likely not the telltale signs of an orgasm but rather the telltale signs that he was irritating her clitoris to the point where she couldn't bear it any longer.

12 THE LOVED ONE

Having just learned the rather strict Ladies First ethic of the First One, Adrian was determined to assist the Loved One to orgasm before he let his penis into the game at all. She very cooperatively had an orgasm the first and every subsequent time he went down on her, so he stuck with head. At first her orgasms were rather violent, on account of his overattention to her clitoris. This rookie error was corrected over the first few weeks of their relationship. With her help, he learned to pay attention to her labia, perineum, and asshole before taking on her clitoris. Her resulting orgasms built more gently to a more satisfying climax.

13 THE GREAT ONE

Adrian tried to help the Great One to orgasm with head and she could have cum that way—she told him as much—but she only had one orgasm in her and always wanted to save that for when his cock was inside her. She liked cumming while filled and could achieve her orgasm quite easily by angling her hips against him.

14 THE LAST ONE

15 THE TALKER

He'd barely started eating her out the first time when he felt something scraping around near his mouth. It was the Talker's nails. The entire time he was down there, she rubbed her clitoris then backed off, ran her finger down the crease between her labia, then drew her hand away, even fucked herself. In between, she'd pet his hair and face, which he found encouraging. She seemed to be having several orgasms—not the heroic, skull-cracking types that the Loved One had, but her body definitely went through cycles of orgasmic tension and relaxation.

Only he didn't half understand what she was up to until they finally fucked. One morning, he'd barely tasted her snatch when she grabbed his ears, pulled his head up to her face and took his cock inside her for the first time.

After a few strokes, he felt something strange. It was her fingers. She was fucking herself right alongside his cock. Then she pulled out and put them in her mouth. That whole time she'd been masturbating with him, she'd been eating her own cum. She'd give herself several more orgasms that way while they fucked.

Adrian came to understand that it wasn't so much that she was having orgasms from anything he was doing and more like she was masturbating while Adrian's face was planted in her box and then again with his cock in there. The whole thing was so crazy nasty that it was more than OK with him.

16 THE ENTHUSIAST

Like the Talker, the Enthusiast seemed to have orgasms while he was going down on her but because of his being almost constantly drunk while they were together, he would be reluctant to put his hand to a holy book about whether she came while they were fucking. She would fuck and suck and be fucked and sucked until Adrian rolled off, then she'd lie beside him and masturbate him with one hand while masturbating herself with the other. This would give her one or two discreet orgasms that Adrian would hardly have noticed either, if it hadn't been for the distinct patterns of breathing and muscular tension that accompanied them.

17 THE EXPERT

Just the opposite of the Great One, the Expert could not cum with Adrian's cock in her snatch. She didn't cum in his mouth, either. They would progress from oral sex to fucking then to ass-fucking. While he was ass-fucking her, she would masturbate to orgasm with a vibrator or just her fingers. Or if the ass-fucking got too intense for her, she'd pull herself off his cock and masturbate while holding on to him.

CHAPTER 6.

Adrian and Your Asshole

Sometime between the first and fifth time in bed with Adrian, you might find yourself wondering, "Why is Adrian playing with my asshole, and what should I do about it?" Excellent question, simple answer: Adrian really enjoys playing with your asshole. In case you haven't thought about what you might or might not let Adrian Colesberry do with your asshole, take some time to do so now.

Things I'd Let Adrian Colesberry Do with My Asshole

1. _____
2. _____
3. _____
4. _____
5. _____
6. _____
7. _____
8. _____
9. _____
10. _____

If you've filled in several of the blanks, good on you. You'll have a wonderful time when Adrian turns his attentions in that direction. But don't panic if your list is short or even blank, he will gently help you move some items onto it.[1] And don't panic about the whole "move some items onto it" thing either. This does not mean that Adrian, on your third time sleeping together, will unfurl onto your bed a velveteen tool-roll filled with a series of butt plugs starting at pinkie size and working up by small increments to the exact diameter of his erect penis. Not at all.

The man would be quite happy if he could just give you rimjobs and massage your asshole with his fingers. There are many women who will accept no more, and Adrian would enjoy making love to all of them. Not to say that he wouldn't be interested in finger-banging your asshole—he would happily demonstrate his aptitude in this department. If you're agreeable, he'd like to see how you enjoyed some kind of ass toy up there. And would he like to fuck you in the ass? Absolutely. He'd love it, but as much as he'd love it, he's just not interested in sacrificing the rest of your relationship to some crass and unsubtle sodomy quest.

It's not that Adrian doesn't care for ass-fucking. He does. Very much.[2] When he finally fucked a woman in the ass, it turned out to be everything he thought it would be. Having said that, you have to understand that he had no unrealistic expectations about it either. He didn't imagine that it would feel like there were a thousand angels up there fellating him.

The ass-denying reader may wonder, "How is he going to love my asshole if I don't let him put his penis inside it?" Because that's just not the way love works. Adrian will love your asshole regardless. Parents love their child who still hasn't quite gotten out of community college (but seriously is just about to get enough credits to transfer to university) just as much as they love their child who's a successful doctor. In the same way, Adrian will love your asshole whether or not it's open for business.

Tip: *If you want to know if Adrian still loves you, don't bother asking him, "Do you still love me?" He's never going to fall for that one. Instead, ask him, "Do you ever think about fucking me in the ass?" If he doesn't light up, you're done.*[3]

CHAPTER 6 NOTES

1   One day early on in their relationship, Adrian started massaging the Great One's asshole. Her body stiffened, then she mentioned good-naturedly but firmly, "By the way, that place where you have your finger right now? You are never going to put your penis in there."

He reassured her that his finger wasn't a scouting party for his penis and that he liked playing with her asshole even without the prospect of fucking it. He promised to stop if she didn't enjoy it, but fortunately that wasn't necessary. She kindly gave him the green light, with the understanding that he would never try to put his penis or even his finger inside her, ever.

You may be disappointed that Adrian didn't use an array of brilliant psychological techniques to maneuver the Great One into ass sex, but he didn't. In the ass-sex department, Adrian is willing to bide his time—and he will bide it in silence.

His fear was that even if he only asked about it once every six months, somewhere in the back of her mind, the Great One would think that everything he did in bed and maybe everything that came out of his mouth was a part of Adrian Colesberry's Five-Year Plan to Sweaty Ass Sex.

With the Great One, he just stayed on the outside with his fingers and tongue, but she never even got used to that. Even after weeks of his playing with her asshole, she jerked around like he was sending two thousand volts through her every time he touched it.

The ass-phobic reader may be saying, "Yes Adrian, she reacted like that because it's nasty." Adrian agrees. It is nasty. That's the magic of ass sex—familiarity doesn't make it any less nasty. This unchanging characteristic makes ass sex a reliable guard against the sexual exchange becoming routine. There's no such thing for Adrian as "Ho-hum, I'm fingering your asshole." It's just too nasty for that.

2   The first and only woman whom Adrian would ass-fuck was the Expert. She hadn't been just talking when she'd bragged about enjoying ass sex. Their first time in bed, he flipped her on her stomach to give her a rimjob. After less than a minute, she blurted out, "My turn!" Then she squirmed out from under him, scrambled like a monkey onto his back, spread his butt-cheeks and shoved her tongue as far as it would go up his ass, which was quite a ways.

She kept at it for a while then did kind of a somersault and ended up underneath him with his cock in her mouth. Once he got hard, she rolled a condom on him, pulled herself up him, and wrapped her legs around his hips. After fucking for just a bit, she pulled him out of her snatch and pushed the head of his cock up against her anus. From then on, ass-fucking became a regular part of their lovemaking, although Adrian made sure they didn't do it every time; that way ass sex could keep its status as a freaky treat.

Considering how marvelously forward she was about lending him her own asshole, the Expert's shyness about her desire to put something up his was positively quaint. After weeks of only giving him the occasional rimjob, the Expert rolled under him in a 69 one afternoon and busted out her real plans. While he fucked her face, she finger-banged him with two or three or it could have been all of her tiny little fingers.

Then the day came when the Expert's vibrator went belly-up. On learning about the tragedy, Adrian took her on a field trip to his favorite sex shop. After picking out her new vibrator, they started looking around for other fun stuff. The Expert quickly located a wall of butt plugs and stared excitedly at the variety on display.

She had established early on that she didn't get off on having pieces of plastic shoved up her ass—"Flesh only, please"—which was fine with Adrian: If his penis and fingers were the two things that she wanted up her ass, he wasn't super-motivated to add competing items to the list.

The Expert was getting all wet not because she wanted Adrian to ass-fuck *her* with any of the toys, but because she wanted to ass-fuck Adrian with them. To make sure he knew what she was after, she pointed to one butt plug and asked, "Are you sure it isn't too big for you?" As she was letting him sodomize her regularly, it seemed inegalitarian in the extreme to turn her down, especially looking at her lost-puppy face. He threw the butt plug in the basket with the vibrator and they packed off for home.

Leading by example, she had him fuck her in the ass for a while then asked if she could break out the butt plug. Overexcited, the Expert made the rookie error of literally fucking Adrian with the butt plug, as opposed to just leaving it once she worked it in there. By the time he called her on it, the misstep had already caused Adrian some discomfort. Embarrassed, the Expert said she was sorry then sucked his cock forever to make up for it.

3 Adrian used to daydream all the time about ass-fucking the Wife. That daydream lasted exactly as long as his hope for their marriage. One day he stopped thinking about fucking her in the ass and, within a year, he was suing for divorce.

Getting Kinky with Adrian Colesberry

Bondage

If you like to have all or a portion of your sex in a condition of restraint, here's where you finally get yours. At the same time, the bondage nonfan needn't be concerned from this section that lovemaking with Adrian Colesberry will, after a brief honeymoon period, consist of your being trussed up for hours while he takes liberties with your immobilized body. You are in control of how frequently Adrian ties you up. If you hate it, he'll pick up on it and he'll drop the bondage. If you love it, be responsive and he'll keep it up . . . play your cards right and you won't get three steps inside the door before he slaps a cuff on you.

Left to his own devices, Adrian will only tie you up as a nasty treat or in an emergency. The emergency being you don't do anything with your hands. It might seem an obvious point, but Adrian likes to feel wanted while fucking. When a woman proves unwilling to make love to him with anything other than her vagina, he feels somewhat unwanted. This will probably not be a problem with you, but if it is, Adrian has a rule that he will apply.

Adrian's Rule: *"If you don't use your hands, I will tie you up."*[1]

You might be saying, "I haven't heard that kind of authority from Adrian before." Maybe it frightens you. Maybe you like it. Maybe it frightens you *and* you like it.

It's wrong to think of "emergency bondage" as a punishment (unless it turns you on to think of it as punishment, in which case it's totally right to think of it as a punishment). It's more a way for Adrian to manage his expectations. If your hands are free and you're not touching his nipples or face or balls, he's likely to feel under-loved, but tying you up solves those problems: When his caress-starved mind wonders, "Why isn't she cupping my balls?" his rational mind points out, "She's not cupping your balls because her hands are manacled to the corners of the bed." And then he feels better about it.

Whichever variety—emergency or nasty fun—it happens to be, Adrian will introduce bondage in the following stepwise manner (each of these steps will play out over one or several encounters):[2]

1. He will hold your hands above your head while you fuck. This is a good gauge of whether you enjoy being in a state of enforced helplessness while getting fucked.
2. If you like the hand-holding, he will faux-tie your wrists with your panties. This is a safe start for everyone. If you freak out, he will act like he was just doing something random and nasty with your panties—no explanation required. And for you, they're a great starter bondage device, because they're your own clothing and something that you could easily tear out of if you wanted to.
3. If you're turned on by the panties, he will broach the topic of bondage by saying something like, "I'd love to tie you up." You can green light this verbally or just by being more physically responsive.
4. He'll go out and get the equipment necessary to tie you up and then tie you up with it.

In this final stage, it's important for you to understand that bondage is an equipment-heavy pastime (and Adrian has the credit-card bills to prove it).[3] To help him not break the bank, please input your answers into the following decision tree.

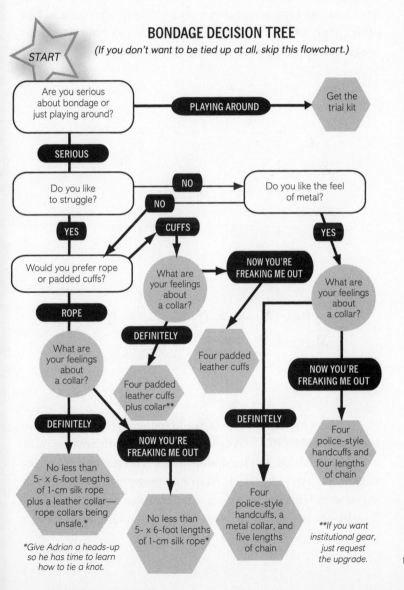

BONDAGE DECISION TREE
(If you don't want to be tied up at all, skip this flowchart.)

START

Are you serious about bondage or just playing around?

PLAYING AROUND → Get the trial kit

SERIOUS

Do you like to struggle? — NO → Do you like the feel of metal?

NO → CUFFS

YES → Would you prefer rope or padded cuffs?

CUFFS → What are your feelings about a collar?

NOW YOU'RE FREAKING ME OUT

YES → What are your feelings about a collar?

ROPE → What are your feelings about a collar?

DEFINITELY → Four padded leather cuffs plus collar**

Four padded leather cuffs

NOW YOU'RE FREAKING ME OUT

DEFINITELY → No less than 5- x 6-foot lengths of 1-cm silk rope plus a leather collar— rope collars being unsafe.*

NOW YOU'RE FREAKING ME OUT

DEFINITELY

NOW YOU'RE FREAKING ME OUT → Four police-style handcuffs and four lengths of chain

*Give Adrian a heads-up so he has time to learn how to tie a knot.

No less than 5- x 6-foot lengths of 1-cm silk rope*

Four police-style handcuffs, a metal collar, and five lengths of chain

**If you want institutional gear, just request the upgrade.

119

This basic equipment allows Adrian to tie you up. But that very phrase "tie you up" raises the question of what to tie you up to. Adrian could construct some kind of dungeon, but unless that's really, seriously your bag, he's more likely to opt for the simpler and more economic solution of running straps between the box spring and the mattress of your bed. Strap arrangement becomes, therefore, a crucial decision that dictates how exactly he can tie you up. The simplest arrangement is as follows:

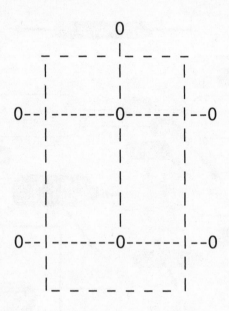

It allows for leg and arm restraint (either to the side or above the head). While this arrangement would be sufficient for most bondage scenarios, Adrian doesn't prefer it on account of its vertical asymmetry: There is no strap at the bottom of the bed. What if you were lying upside down and he wanted to tie your hands directly above your head? And there's no option at all for the corners.

Bondage doesn't petrify Adrian because of its potentially creepy, dungeony aspects, but for the same reason that any costumey perversion is scary: There's no easy out. Say he tries to put you into some laugh-worthy circus position or he flops your arm over his cock and starts to fuck your armpit. If you act like he's just farted at a wedding, no big deal. He can laugh it off, like he was only joking, and transition back into something safe. But if he drags out four faux-fur-lined leather cuffs with a not-matching but also faux-fur-lined leather collar and clips them to straps that he's run beneath his mattress, there's no shrugging it off. None of that could have happened by accident.[4]

It may seem like overkill, but here's a strap arrangement that provides the versatile restraint required by Adrian Colesberry.

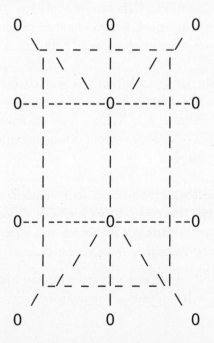

Make copies of the previous page and use a marker to draw your limbs onto the bed schematic. How would you like to be tied up? At the corners for the classic X? Hands straight up and feet to the side? Use your imagination. And if you like, draw some positions you'd bind Adrian into.

No one has ever done so, but perhaps you could tie him up and sit on his face. That can't miss. Or if you really want to teach him a thing or two, tie him up and make him watch you masturbate.

The Struggle

You'll have noticed that the equipment choice relies a lot on whether you're planning to struggle or whether you're just going to lie there while he fucks you. Having studied your response with the panties and the wrist-holding, Adrian will be able to make an educated guess on this topic, but you should be aware of what you like. All things being equal, Adrian would prefer some struggling on your part—not too much or you'll both be too tired to fuck after.

Fortunately for you, Adrian has worked out an energy-conserving, partly choreographed wrestling match that you can step through whenever you decide to play the bondage game. It gives the illusion of struggle without exhausting either or both of you into uselessness. [5]

> *Step 1.* He'll wrestle you onto your stomach, straddle your back, and pin your arms under his knees. Once he's got you trapped, you can struggle as much as you want. In that position, he puts the collar around your neck.

> *Step 2.* He'll release one arm at a time and buckle the cuffs onto your wrists. If your wrists and hands are small, this will

be the hard step. Unless he gets it on the tightest possible notch, you'll be able to slip right out.

Step 3. He'll clip both of your wrists to the collar. At the end of this move, you'll be done up top.

Step 4. He'll flip himself around and get your feet. It's really important that you don't struggle too much with your legs because you might kick his teeth out. He'll attach cuffs to your ankles and then clip them to the straps at the sides or corners of the bed.

Step 5. One at a time, he'll unclip your wrists from the collar and attach them to the straps.

Done, and plenty of gas left in the tank![6]

Aggression

For Adrian Colesberry, lust feels a lot like aggression. He's been aware of this for many years, so he's not going to get confused, like teenage boys often do, and say something mean when he really wants to touch your boobs. He'll just touch your boobs (if and only if that's already a part of your relationship). That way, you don't get your feelings hurt and you do get your boobs touched. Win-win.

Once you start fucking him, you might think that his feelings of lust would clarify themselves, seeing as they are being directly addressed, but just the opposite is the case: They get closer and closer to aggression, in an asymptotic approach. Again, he's in control of this and isn't liable to get confused and insult your mother when he likes your mother fine but wants to flip you into doggie-style. He'll just flip you into doggie-style without a word about your mother. And assuming that you enjoy getting vigorously fucked from behind, that's another win for the both of you.

Over the years, Adrian has learned to channel his lust/aggression in various ways that make it not a burden on your lovemaking but a benefit.

Fucking super-hard

Most often, when he feels his aggression welling up, Adrian will take it out on you with his penis by upping his pump speed. This usually takes the stuffing out of him for the moment and works for you, too, hopefully.

Dirty-talking

When dirty-talking, Adrian's aggression comes out in his tone of voice, not in the content. As emphasized previously, he's not going to say anything mean.

Playing with your asshole

Needless to say, Adrian will never play with your asshole in an aggressive manner. It just feels aggressive to play with your asshole at all, even in the gentle, skilled idiom employed by Adrian Colesberry.

Hair-pulling

In a hyperaggressive variation on pinning your hands above your head, Adrian can use your hair to pin your head to the mattress while fucking you.[7] In case you've never had your hair pulled in an erotic context, it's not painful, catfight hair-pulling—no yanking or tearing involved. Done properly, Adrian gets so much of your hair in his fist that regardless of how hard he pulls, the force is evenly distributed and never triggers the pain threshold of any particular strand. It's the same physics principle that allows a yogi to comfortably distribute his or her weight across a bed of nails. In the case of hair-pulling, the force of the pull is distributed across hairs instead of weight across nails. The possibility of pain is tantalizingly imminent but never happens.

Struggling/Bondage

If you're kind enough to struggle through the position changes, Adrian can put his aggression into that. If you like getting tied up, especially if you're into struggling against the bonds, that'll work too.

Spanking

Remember back when you learned how much Adrian liked to smack you on the ass? How you were promised that letting him do it wouldn't open the door to any kind of spanking or punishment thing? Do not now come to the conclusion that those promises are being broken and that his supposedly innocent smack on the ass does inevitably invite the spanking. It doesn't.

True, Adrian would very much like to direct his aggression into some kind of spanking, punishment thing, but he'll have wanted to do this regardless of whether you let him smack you on the ass.[8] You might enjoy a spanking while he fucks you doggie-style. He'll enjoy spanking you while you suck his cock because, to Adrian, this seems ungrateful and ungentlemanly in the extreme and therefore very aggressive. When he feels particularly angry, he might grab your hair, pin your head to the mattress, spank you for a run, then fuck you from behind. And every once in a while, you might enjoy throwing yourself across his lap so he can spank you like some angry daddy punishing his little girl.

As always, you are in control. If he keeps going after you want him to stop, say "stop" or "fuck me" or "don't." If he's throwing too heavy a hand, say "ouch" or something like that and he'll back off. You can consider any of those, or their synonyms, to be your safe words.

Spanking is the first of these aggression-oriented activities where it helps for you to like a little pain. The reader who doesn't like the pain is not going to enjoy a spanking. Adrian is particularly sensitive to this factor because he doesn't like the pain himself and as a result doesn't particularly enjoy a spanking.

Nonetheless, if Adrian's spanking you, he'll certainly let you spank him. Fair is fair. You should know that it won't do any good for his erection and will send his already reluctant orgasm into an all but total retreat. But if you're willing to go to heroic efforts to get his erection back after a spanking, knock yourself out. Maybe your heroics will be such a mind-blowing kink-fest that he'll learn to like a spanking after all.

Paddling

From the beginning of his spanking career, Adrian harbored a prejudice against spanking aids in favor of the more intimate, less sadistic-seeming spanking by hand. But as Adrian learned, and as the experienced already know, if spanking goes beyond a few minutes, the paddle is a kindness. The kindness of the paddle is dictated by the same physics principle just encountered that allows hair to be pulled without any pain: distribution of force over area.

The surface area of Adrian Colesberry's hand is approximately 25.3 inches square. This might sound large, but it's pretty normal. A credit card has an area of 7.8 inches square, so it's just a bit more than the area of three credit cards put together. A normal size for a paddle is 5 inches by 9 inches, giving a surface area of 45 inches square—nearly double that of Adrian's hand. Say Adrian swings both the paddle and his hand with a force of 20 pounds. (This number wasn't pulled out of the sky but measured by having Adrian spank an analog bathroom scale and observing the highest reach of the needle. The highest reach observed was 12 pounds, but this number was adjusted upward by two-thirds in consideration of the inertial elements inside the scale, which would low-bias its measurement of an instantaneous impact force.) At 20 pounds, his hand would strike your ass with an impact (expressed in pressure units) of 0.79 pounds per square inch (psi), whereas the paddle would strike at 0.44 psi.

On top of this nearly 50 percent reduction in impact, the paddle handle is flexible (unlike the bones in Adrian's forearm) setting a limit on the maximum impact. These built-in safety factors eliminate the bruising and lingering soreness that can result from overzealous spanking. So don't freak out when Adrian introduces the paddle. He's not on the road to building a dungeon; he's noted your enjoyment of spanking and he feels that you'll be more safely satisfied with the paddle than with his hand.[9]

Face-slapping

Even if you like the tying up and the spanking and the hair-pulling and everything else that comes along with Adrian's aggressive lovemaking style, it may still make you angry the first time he slaps you in the face. To Adrian, that's the good news because mainly he's slapping you in the face so you'll slap him back.

The psychodynamically oriented reader might have anticipated Adrian's need for physical reprisal. Yes, it could be that part of his psyche is uncomfortable with his aggressive fucking style and wants you to dish out a little in his direction, or maybe he's playing out some nonconsensual sex fantasy—probably a bit of both. Whatever it is, he won't be able to come out and ask you to slap him. He isn't good in that area.

To Adrian's brain, a slap in the face is so offensive that if he slaps you, you won't have any choice but to slap him back. He'll figure this even if you don't spank him back or pull his hair back or tell him that he's nasty back. Those things he will consider part of the hypermasculine/hyperfeminine game that you play on occasion. But the personal affront that is a slap in the face doesn't fit comfortably into that category so demands a different response—at least he hopes so.[10]

Perhaps you do not want Adrian to slap you at all but would still like to try slapping him. That'll be fine. Just go for it. Missionary's the best position. Concentrate on slapping him on the face and chest while he's fucking you. You could try backhanding him from doggie-style, but that seems like a formula for a broken tooth.

Role-playing

The detail-oriented reader might object to the appearance of role-playing in this context since not every scenario would provide an outlet for Adrian's aggression. Very true. For example, if you say, "Nice doggie," he'll bark or whine a bit, sniff you all over, and give you a rimjob. If you say, "Beauregard, I do believe I've turned my ankle," he'll adopt a Southern accent, carry you around the house until you indicate that you'd like to be set down, then he'll make love to your feet. No aggression required.

But the critical advantage of role-playing is well illustrated in both of these examples: Note how you were able to direct Adrian's behavior with great specificity without coming right out and directing his behavior. This confers an advantage for several reasons: First off, if you're constantly barking out instructions, Adrian's going to start feeling more like your masseur than your lover. Second, when it comes to the aggressive stuff, even the reader who very much wants a spanking may not want to ask for one directly. Much like it's impossible to tickle yourself, it may be difficult for you to enjoy a spanking that you've asked for.

Third and most important, if you've found out that the pain is what you're after, it's imperative to establish some context in which it makes sense for Adrian to be spanking/paddling you for a long time. You might be thinking, "Why? I don't need any context!" It's fine if you don't, but Adrian definitely does.

Left to his own devices, Adrian will spank you to turn himself on, which takes a couple of minutes max, then he'll fuck you until he needs to recharge, spank you until he gets hard again, then recommence the fucking and on and on. If this isn't what you're interested in, if you want Adrian to roll up his sleeves and spank your ass scarlet, definitely work with him to find a plausible excuse. For example, you can be a prisoner or a slave girl.[11]

One limitation on this one: Your slave girl cannot be located in the pre–Civil War American South. Adrian is a Southern man. There is nothing remotely erotic to him about playing master/slave if he is the master of an American slave of African descent. That sits way too close to the appalling historical reality of his little corner of the world for it to give him a hard-on. Although this scenario is especially nasty, even Adrian has limits.

You don't ever have to get specific with the era or ethnicity, but if you do, it's best to locate your slave girl deep in the safety of classical history. That's what Adrian does inside his head. If you say nothing, you'll be the daughter of a shipwrecked Phoenician ship captain and he'll be a Greek farmer living on the coast of Asia Minor who has to punish you like this because you're always trying to escape. But no matter how much he beats you, he can never break your spirit. That kind of thing.

For the reader who sees Adrian's inability to beat a fantasy Southern slave as yet another opportunity denied women of color, do please forgive the man, he's not perfect, as you must by now have realized.

CHAPTER 7 NOTES

1   One night, a few weeks into their relationship, Adrian found himself holding the Innocent One's hands above her head while they fucked. He let go as soon as he noticed. But she left her wrists crossed above her head on the pillow as if he had never released them. He kept fucking her and she kept not moving them, so finally, he allowed himself to hold them again.

After realizing what he was up to, Adrian subtly planted a thought in the Innocent One's head: "I don't know what it is, but when we make love I feel like . . . tying you up or something." She kissed him a little harder. Good. He was on the right track. It was at this moment that Adrian formulated his famous rule, "If you don't use your hands, I will tie you up." Adrian took a trip to his favorite sex shop but didn't see anything that the Innocent One would find friendly enough. Their relationship ended before he got around to tying her up.

2   In the case of the Great One, Adrian bypassed this sequence because she brought it up herself. One day, out of the blue, a few weeks after he had graciously accepted the fact that he would never put his cock in her ass, the Great One said, "I'm not going to try anal sex, but I'm totally open to anything else."* Then she tacked on an example of what "anything else" meant. "Like, you could tie me up or something." Easy to see why he didn't interpret this as her own personal desire to get tied up.

He didn't need a concession prize for not crassly trying to fuck her in the ass every weekend, so Adrian let the remark pass unacknowledged. But later that week, it dawned on him that if she thought she was denying him something by withholding ass sex and if she thought that she could make up for it by letting him tie her up, what kind of inconsiderate boor was he to deprive her of her ability to make up for it, even if he didn't think there was anything to make up for?

3   At Adrian's favorite sex shop, a sexy tattooed saleslady who borrowed her basic moves from the stereo salesman sold him all his bondage equipment. But hers wasn't just a cynical sales pitch; she genuinely educated Adrian about what he should expect from the bondage experience—an education that you too can benefit from.

---

* The following point cannot, apparently, be emphasized enough: Your asshole is not a door. By logical extension, when he touches your asshole, Adrian is not knocking for you to open it up for him. If you insist on thinking about your asshole in this way, his persistent interest in playing with it might make you think, as the Great One did, that he's feeling deprived and that everything he does to your asshole is him pressuring you to let his penis in there. Not so. He understands that he won't be putting his penis in every one of your body's orifices. If he kisses your ear, it's not a prelude to his trying to finger-bang your ear hole. Same with your anus. So there's no need to build up a defensive position by countering ass sex with other high-profile perversions.

Step #1. Set the Educative Tone

She started by detailing the pros and cons of the various methods of bondage. Police-style handcuffs are for people who like the feel of the metal, but not for someone who likes to struggle, because the metal can cut and bruise. She showed him several varieties of padded cuffs that allowed the bonded to struggle in luxurious comfort. Rope also allows for struggling but requires a lot of tying and untying, so you have to know a few knots. From this information, Adrian decided that he wanted the Great One to be able to struggle and, since he couldn't tie a knot, he'd have to go with the padded cuffs.

Step #2. Ridicule the Low-End

Once he'd chosen the kind of equipment he wanted, the sexy saleslady walked him to the front of the store where they had the novelty items—pencils with boobs for erasers and things like that. Pointing to a selection of bondage starter kits, she confided to him that she encouraged fly-by-night experimenters to get an inexpensive, leopard-print, nylon set—perfect for folks who want a naughty Valentine's Day gift that will be unwrapped, played with until someone starts giggling, then stuffed into a drawer never to emerge again. The cheap kits are comfortable enough for struggling, just not durable.

The saleslady said, with a hint of a challenge, "If you aren't sure that your partner will like it, you should probably just get the kit."

No, Adrian would not be skulking out with the cheap, leopard-print, nylon bondage kit.

Step #3. Dismiss Fears of Over-Buying by Trotting Out the Ultra–High-End

The sexy saleslady suggested that for anybody serious about bondage—by now this was totally Adrian Colesberry—only faux-fur-lined, leather cuffs would do. He completely agreed.

When he flinched at the cost, she ignored his reaction and continued showing him the various styles—making pains to point out some super-padded, double-buckled tan leather cuffs that cost five times the amount of the ones she was trying to sell him. "These are the cuffs they use in insane asylums. You can struggle as much as you want without hurting yourself. . . . But you don't need these."

Adrian thought, "No, that's right. I don't need those. She under-stands me."

Enthusiastic reader, perhaps Adrian has profoundly underes-timated your needs here. If you require insane asylum–style re-straints attached to half-inch-thick eyebolts screwed directly into the wall beams . . . by all means, he'll get a second job and rethink his equipment choice. He'll buy a straightjacket and pad a small room.

Step #4. Enhance the Prospect's Perceived Need

"Do you need to restrain just the hands or the feet, too?" He'd only ever thought to restrain the Great One's hands, but now that she mentioned the feet. . . . "It's not like you have to do it every time, but if you don't have the cuffs, you don't have the option to do it." Bondage options! That's exactly what Adrian needed. Yes, he absolutely had to be able to restrain her feet.

Finally he climbed off the fence and chose a set of four black-patent-leather, faux-fur-lined cuffs.

Step #5. Uncover Hidden Needs

The saleslady asked, "Do you need a collar?" The idea of put-ting a collar on the Great One seemed more a humiliation tactic than an absolutely necessary step to immobilize her limbs, and he said so. But wait. His saleslady explained patiently that it wasn't only for that.

With some two-sided metal clips, he could hook both her wrist cuffs to the ring at the front of the collar. Then she'd be re-strained but he could still move her from place to place. Plus, when she was sucking his cock, her hands would be perfectly positioned near her mouth to help out.

With this explanation, the saleslady had climbed inside Adrian's brain. He longed for the restrained but blowjob-efficient woman. Clearly, he needed the collar most of all. What else had he even gone in there for?

Finally, he walked out, his wallet much lighter, carrying enough equipment to satisfy any beginning bondage connoisseur. He had four matching faux-fur-lined, patent-leather cuffs, inter-changeable for either ankles or wrists; a non-matching—with his saleslady's apologies—faux-fur-lined, leather collar; several pairs of straps for under the bed; an assortment of double-sided, quick-release clips and some metal rings, to allow for flexibility of configuration, because Adrian Colesberry needed flexibility of configuration.

4   Adrian was particularly worried about getting the cuffs on the Great One while she sat there watching him. That's why, before heading down to her place, he stopped to get one more piece of equipment—a blindfold. (You don't have to weigh in on whether you want a blindfold. It's not for you. It's for Adrian.)

They fucked normal first, then during a break, Adrian unceremoniously dumped all the stuff on the bed. She handled the different pieces for a while. Once her curiosity was satisfied, he put the blindfold on her and started fitting her with the collar. It was kind of tricky because of all her hair, but the blindfold transformed his incompetent fumbling into a deliberately slow, sensual process.

He attached her wrists to the collar and, immediately, she folded her arms against her chest like a wounded bird. Then, as they fucked, she played the cold, hard metal rings against her breasts, face, and mouth. For the Great One, he should have bought the police cuffs.

She seemed to be enjoying herself, which made him happy, but she was so different tied up than free that, ultimately, he missed her being free and unhitched her. She never stayed tied up for long.

5   As much as Adrian loves the struggle, it's important to understand that he doesn't need to legitimately overpower you. First of all, he probably can't, not without hurting you or, more likely, you hurting him. At any moment, you'll be able to end the charade by flipping over or jerking your hand out of his grip or kneeing him in the testicles. As you know, his are very sensitive, so that'll do the trick for sure.

However, don't let this frank evaluation of Adrian's physical abilities make you think that you'll be doing the acting job of your life in letting him overpower you. Not at all. He's a reasonably strong guy to whom many people wouldn't be embarrassed to lose a wrestling match.

And since the whole thing's a game, you can take a turn as the victor if you'd like. Adrian will be happy to lose as long as you take the responsibility belonging to the winner: giving the loser head for a long spell then fucking their brains out.

6   The Kind One would struggle against the cuffs the entire time she was in them. For her, there was no such thing as "Fine, I'll sit here while you tie me up." It ruined her experience to cooperate. Just like he needed to feel her pushback, she needed to feel his weight, the strength of his muscles overpowering hers.

And even though the woman only played at resisting, she played pretty hard. The first few times he tied her up, it took so much out of him that he was dripping sweat by the time the final cuff was clipped to the final strap.

One time, she struggled so much that he pooped out after getting only her wrists strapped in—not to the straps at the corners but the ones on the sides of the bed. She pushed up onto her knees, at which point he thought she wanted to be fucked doggie-style, but that wasn't it. She kept working her knees underneath her body and, even though he'd made the straps super-tight, continued to pull until she got all the way up into a kneeling position and flattened herself against the wall at the head of his bed.

With her arms stretched to their limit, she started bouncing up and down on the mattress, scraping her breasts against the wall. Bounce, bounce, bounce. After a few minutes, the Kind One started pouring sweat. Still, it seemed that she'd never tire out. Adrian started giving her a handjob, only this had a calming effect that she didn't like at all. She squirmed away from his fingers. OK, no handjob. But he wanted her to stay with him somehow so, thinking on his feet, he put a finger up her ass. That worked. She started moving furiously again. Finally, exhausted, she withered against the wall and he unhitched her.

Both of them were too tired to fuck after that. This bondage stuff was not working out . . . yet. You'll be happy to know that they didn't give up. Over their next several evenings together, Adrian and the Kind One would come up with the five-step choreographed bondage sequence that Adrian uses to this day.

7   One afternoon in bed, Adrian was losing his erection when, either by accident or by instinct, he took his free hand and grabbed a fistful of the Great One's long, curly, dark hair, right near the scalp, and pinned her head to the mattress. In the time it took him to perform the action, he got completely hard again.

Adrian noticed the change in his arousal but didn't immediately accept the connection between his level of aggression and his hard-on. Historically, he had always, only, and ever been a sweet lover. (Even when holding the Innocent One's hands above her head, he had done so in the most tender way possible.) It made him feel ungentlemanly to be pulling the Great One's hair, so he let up after a bit. When he did, his hard-on immediately backed off to semierect. Once he grabbed for her hair again, it just as immediately returned. After a few cycles with the same results, he could no longer avoid the conclusion that grabbing her hair was turning him on.

Note how Adrian is a reflexive experimenter. In a new situation (like hair-pulling), he automatically establishes a control (no hair-pulling) and then tries different variations in position or speed or force or whatever to determine exactly what is causing the observed effect (his erection). You probably wouldn't notice in the moment, and even if you became conscious of his switching stuff back and forth, you probably wouldn't perceive it as an experiment but as a man expressing his passion for variety. But if you ever do catch on that he's conducting some kind of experiment and it's killing your buzz, just tell him to cut it out. He can get back to the lab later.

Even after he proved to himself that the hair-pulling was the only thing keeping him hard, he probably wouldn't have kept it up, except the Great One seemed to be loving it. During a break, she said, delighted, "Wow! I didn't expect that from you." He laughed, happy that she was enjoying herself. It had surprised him much more than it possibly could have surprised her.

8 Several weeks after the hair-pulling incident, Adrian and the Great One were midway through an afternoon of fucking when she pitched herself over his lap and half-commanded, half-pleaded, "Spank me!"

He'd never spanked a girl (maybe since his parents never spanked Baby Adrian, it just wasn't lodged in his brain as some erotic potential waiting to be realized), so her request caught him entirely flat-footed. They'd never talked about spanking or punishment, but he had been unusually aggressive with the Great One—unusual that is for him—so it's easy to see how she thought that a request for him to spank her would be warmly welcomed.

He looked down, totally in shock, at her beautiful ass cheeks— ass cheeks that Adrian Colesberry had fondled, squeezed, stroked, kissed, licked, segmented like an orange to get at her sweet, equally kissable little asshole, but never even once considered spanking.

The Great One had buried her head in the mattress—that curly, black hair covering every inch of her face. No help from a playful glance. He was on his own.

Hard to know exactly how much time had passed from the time she asked him . . . maybe four seconds . . . before he started paddling the tar out of her. No, he did *not* start out timidly and ramp up. Adrian Colesberry is a people pleaser. The Great One wanted him to spank her, so she got a shellacking.

It might alarm the reader that he would start out spanking so hard. Considering his lack of spanking experience, wouldn't it make more sense for Adrian to start out soft and then increase the intensity? Seems like it, but if you do a quick thought experiment, you'll see that his instinct to start out harder was right.

Imagine you've screwed up your courage to ask Adrian for a spanking—not an easy thing to do, even for the intrepid Great One—and he starts out spanking you too soft. Now what are your options? Either you screw up your courage again and ask him to spank you harder, risking even more than you did the first time that he'll think you're some freaky masochist (not that he wouldn't enjoy your being a freaky masochist, just that you might not want him thinking that). Or you endure his tepid spanking, not getting out of it anything that you wanted, until finally, you get so bored that you lie to him that he's done enough.

But if Adrian starts spanking you too hard, you don't have to say anything to tone things down aside from "ouch." And if you don't even want to say that you can just put your hand over your ass and block him. Either way, he'll get the message and back off.

There does turn out to be a problem with starting out hard, only it's not on the receiver's side. Within a couple of minutes flailing away at the Great One's ass, Adrian's arm started to get tired. He talked himself into thinking of it as an upper-body workout and kept up his efforts, but as the ache in his shoulder turned into a sharp pain, he found himself in a pickle. He briefly considered having her flip around so he could switch to left-handed spanking for a bit, then immediately rejected the idea. He didn't know all the rules to this spanking thing yet, but he was pretty sure that the only person allowed to say, "This hurts. We have to switch sides," was the person getting spanked.

His mind raced around for solutions, but before he could find one, he ran out of time—his arm just gave out at the end of one swing. He stared at his hand resting uselessly on her ass. Then, in this moment of abject failure, the solution came to him—he could extend his still-functional fingers between her legs and finger-fuck her.

When he reached down, her snatch was raining onto the sheets. Inspired by the results of his efforts, his arm recovered quickly. He spanked her then rested in her hole then spanked her some more, until, as quickly as she had requested the spanking, the Great One flipped over onto her back and pulled him inside her.

This is how you remain completely in control of this situation. Stop the spanking at will by inviting Adrian to fuck—something he'll never refuse.

9 One night, Adrian and the Kind One had both had a bit to drink beforehand. And while he was spanking her, she started popping off with stuff like, "I can't even feel that!" and "You wimp!" So he obligingly hit her harder and harder.

Whenever he let up, she'd chastise him for treating her like a porcelain doll: "I'm not going to break! I can take it." He spent more time spanking her than fucking her that night, because she seemed to be enjoying the spanking most and, frankly, he didn't have the energy to do both.

The next morning, he woke abruptly to the Kind One crying out, "Oh, no!" from the bathroom. He knew immediately that he'd made marks and begged her to show him. Reluctantly, she emerged and lay down on the bed. Her entire right ass cheek was a massive, multicolored bruise. Judging from the damage done, he might as well have been punching her with his fist. He felt like crying. She said it was no big deal and dared him to give her just one more whack for good luck. He couldn't.

Tip: Don't get spanked drunk and don't taunt Adrian to spank you harder when he is drunk.

Adrian went to his sex shop and got the largest leather paddle they carried. Nothing fancy. Just two pieces of leather sewn together with a semi-stiff something in the middle so it wouldn't bend in the breeze. Then he put it in a drawer, never even telling her it was there.

For weeks after the bruising incident, every time the Kind One walked through his door, she would pull down her pants and show him her ass—he had sworn off spanking her until the bruise had disappeared. One happy day, it had faded to the point where he felt like he was being mean to hold out on her any longer. After hearing his verdict on the fitness of her ass cheeks, the Kind One threw herself facedown on the bed and demanded a spanking. Adrian took the paddle out of the drawer where he'd been hiding it and gave it to her for examination.

He went at her for a good while and as soon as they woke up the next morning, he flipped her on her stomach to search her ass for bruises. He could only see a couple of faint marks from the edge of the paddle. Making a mental note to keep it absolutely flat to the surface of her ass, he announced that the paddle had passed the test.

Adrian's unwillingness to leave marks might be a deal-breaker for the reader who wants to carry the evidence of a righteous spanking or paddling or whatever you're into. "If he's not going to leave me something to remember him by, I don't know why I'd let him punish me at all." Hold on. That's crazy! All you have to do in this case is inform Adrian about your needs: He'll adjust his goal from "leave no marks" to "definitely leave marks" and you will, guaranteed, get the souvenir(s) you're looking for.

10 After getting slapped in the face for the first time, the Great One said to Adrian in an I've-never-been-to-Paris tone of voice, "No one has ever slapped me like that!" Good, it had turned her on. Not so good, she'd immediately filed face-slapping under Aggressive Things Adrian Does to the Great One That the Great One Does Not Do Back to Adrian. She'd only ever been physically submissive in the face of all his other aggression—not even struggling when he tied her up—so he was hardly surprised. You cannot get all from the same woman. And who'd want to?

Only with the Kind One did he finally get what he wanted from the face-slapping. As he imported all the things he'd learned to enjoy with the Great One, the Kind One had gone with the flow so easily that he assumed she'd done it all before with other boyfriends. So when she mentioned on a break that no one had ever slapped her in the face, he backtracked over all the rest and was surprised to learn that, despite her even-keeled reactions, she'd never been spanked or tied up or had her hair pulled . . .

Nor, she informed him, had anyone put her whole foot in his mouth. This surprised him more than the rest because, although of completely average height, she had the sweetest little morsel of a foot he'd ever seen. Demurely footed reader, do come to bed with clean feet, as much as that's practicable. If Adrian can fit your whole foot in his mouth, he will. That's his circus trick for you.

Once it was out of the bag that all this aggression stuff was totally new to her, Adrian asked the Kind One about each little thing one by one, like polling jurors about a verdict, just to make sure she liked them and wasn't suffering through to get to the parts of the sex she did enjoy. When he got to the face-slapping, the Kind One admitted, "That makes me a little angry!"

Adrian said, "Oh, good!" and suggested that she could slap him back. By then, all the talk had made them both furiously horny, so they went back to it. A few strokes in, the Kind One took him up on his offer, swinging her hand in an arc from her side and cracking him hard in the jaw. Ouch! Well, he'd wanted someone to hit him back.

He started to show her how to control her swing so its force was concentrated on the fleshy parts of his cheek, but she cut him off, saying, "You hit me in the ear!" by which she meant, "If you can't take it, don't dish it out!" Good point.

During sex, slapping the Kind One's sweet, sweet face seemed rude enough, but there was something brutally, unforgivably offensive about slapping her when she was sucking his cock. Adrian even offended himself. But if you think this offensiveness is why it didn't work out, you're on the wrong track. That was the fun part.

The problem came when the Kind One tried to return the favor while he was eating her box. She found herself at a geographical disadvantage here, since her cheeks were out in the open with her mouth around his cock while his cheeks were inaccessibly sandwiched between her thighs when he was going down on her. In an effort to find a substitute, she just banged the flat of her hand on his head. It hurt, but he appreciated it anyway. It's the thought that counts.

11 After the Kind One announced that she didn't want to be called a whore, Adrian became quite gun shy about saying anything. Only his muteness was also a big problem for the Kind One, who had liked his aggressive chatter, but just wanted him to delete the one part of his vocabulary. To give him permission to start talking again, she needed to invent something new for him to say.

One Saturday, they were house-sitting for a friend of hers and had just finished cleaning the dishes from dinner when he mashed her hips against her friend's kitchen counter and started kissing her. He pulled her pants and underwear around her ankles, but just when he was fixing to heave her up onto the counter, she spun around and pushed her bare ass back into him, demanding, "Find something." He opened every drawer within reach, showing her the contents of each. She violently shook her head at the kitchen towels and spatulas until, finally, he grabbed a long-handled wooden spoon. On seeing it she said, "Mmm" and lifted her ass in the air.

He flipped the spoon so that he was holding the head in his hand, grabbed a fistful of her hair, laid out her torso flat across the cold countertop, and gave her ass a whack with the long wooden handle.

"MMM!"

He whacked her a few more times, then again started to take his cock out, but she objected, "Mmm." That's when she let him in on what the game was—in a Mexican accent, she said, "Maria so sorry kitchen isn't clean enough."*

Although he's a bit too self-conscious to invent elaborate bedroom games like this one, Adrian will reward you for putting forward one of your own by jumping on board with all speed. If you walk into the room dressed like a rabbit or a New Orleans hooker or a pirate, he won't stupidly ask why you're dressed funny. He'll catch on immediately that you're a rabbit or a New Orleans hooker or a pirate who wants to be fucked, and will construct a scenario where he'd fuck a rabbit or a New Orleans hooker or a pirate.

---

* If you find the social realism of the Mexican maid too distracting, you could be an Estonian maid. If playing around with any ethnic divide, however obscure, is distasteful to you, go back in time and be a Victorian-era maid. Or if the concept of class domination throws you, maybe you could be a communist worker reporting to a comrade that you didn't make your razor blade quota. Alternately, flip the power relationship and be a CEO caught at corporate fraud by a lowly accountant within your own organization. Point being, you can frame this interaction any way you want.

Adrian reopened the drawer where he'd found the towels and hot-mitts and dug around for an apron. He raised her off the counter by her hair, pulled the apron over her head, and cinched it over-tightly around her waist. He's not so quick on the uptake but once Adrian catches onto something, he does commit.

Retaking a clump of her hair, he pushed her back over the counter and started on her ass with the spoon again. "You think I pay you to mess things up, Maria?!"

Still in character, she whimpered, "No."

He pulled her up, dragged her a few drawers down the counter, and shoved her face within an inch of the still dripping dishes. "You call these clean?!"

"I say I sorry."

He got angrier. "Sometimes sorry isn't good enough, Maria."

She cried, "Oh, no. Please."

Suddenly, the Kind One kicked her pants off her ankles, broke away, and ran out of the kitchen into the dining room. He followed her, curious about what game they were playing next, but when he got there she was gone. He heard her bare feet pattering on the hall floor going back toward the kitchen.

She wasn't going anywhere; she just wanted him to chase her. So he did—every time she looked back at him, he'd wave the spoon threateningly above his head and she'd yelp and run faster.

Eventually, he caught her in the dining room, plopped into an overstuffed chair and started to bend her over the cushiony arm to restart Maria's punishment for the horrible dirty, dirty kitchen, but she fell from the arm onto her knees with a pathetic, "Oh, boss, I sorry." Then she took his cock out of his pants and gave him a blowjob. After that they just fucked—no more accents, no more angry boss.

Regardless of the ethnic, social, or political details, this game plays out in more or less the same way. Adrian punishes you for something; when you've had enough of that, play chase if you want, then blow him to put a stop to the angry portion of the game so he can fuck you sweetly for the rest of the evening.

As he caught on faster and faster, she did that kind of thing more and more—invented a game right off the top of her head, played it through, and then dropped it. She expected him to drop it too, which he did. Maria the Mexican maid? He never saw her again. The next game was different and the next and the next.

The inventive reader might wonder if there are games Adrian won't play. Yes, there are. One time, the Kind One started talking to him in a little girly voice. This had potential until she turned out to be a Catholic schoolgirl. Not a high school girl either—a grade school girl. And he was a child molester who'd picked her up at recess. Just in case you thought it was always a winner to play the Catholic schoolgirl . . . it's not. Adrian heroically tried to play along, but no way was he going to get an erection. She tried to get him to spank her for running away, but he couldn't. He managed to finger-bang her for a while but even that made him sick once she started complaining about the tummy-ache she'd gotten from all the candy he gave her. (Don't believe that for a second. He didn't give her any candy.)

CHAPTER 8

Putting It All Together with Adrian Colesberry

Generous reader, having learned this much about how to make love to Adrian Colesberry, you may be worrying, "It could be that I'm just not enough for him. If I'm not into everything he's into, will I be able to make him happy?" Stop doing that to yourself. You don't have to be everything for Adrian; Adrian won't be everything for you. It's wonderful that you care so much, but you'll be relieved to know that making Adrian happy can be accomplished by following a simple four-step process:

1. Pick your items from his menu.
2. Find a spot for yourself on his pyramid.
3. Keep the experimentation going.
4. Arbitrate any differences that come up using his simple negotiation system.

The Menu

Adrian will import into your relationship all the spanking and the skull-fucking and the playing with your asshole and the bondage and the rest, but while you will end up sampling every item on the menu, he won't expect you to like each dish. It'd be weird if you did. Use positive feedback to keep Adrian serving up what you do enjoy and when a particular item isn't to your taste, just let him know and he'll take it off the menu. (If you want to be clever about things, for every item you take off the menu, replace it with something equally entertaining.)[1]

You'll have menu items of your own, no doubt, so feel free to throw them on the table. A woman bringing ideas into bed is pretty sexy on its own, so Adrian will be highly motivated to figure out a way of enjoying whatever you contribute.

Making Adrian Happy: The Pyramid

All research shows that as long as Adrian Colesberry can go down on you, get a little head back every once in a while, and fuck you in a reasonable variety of positions, he's going to be satisfied with your sex life. But if satisfied isn't good enough for you (an attitude that Adrian would both applaud and reciprocate) there are three things you can do to push him from satisfied up to happy:

1. Suck his cock in an unsolicited, enthusiastic manner.
2. Enjoy/encourage his attentions to your asshole.
3. Enjoy/encourage a spanking or some other form of punishment.

The good news? He doesn't need all three. You can make him ecstatically happy by seriously punching in with only one of these areas or by checking in at a lower level with a combination of two or three of them. The mathematical relationship is best represented on a three-dimensional, pyramid graph.

The graph is shown in top, side, and cutaway views. To envision the zones in three dimensions, imagine them as tightly nested wooden bowls that have been sawed into the shape of a three-sided pyramid.

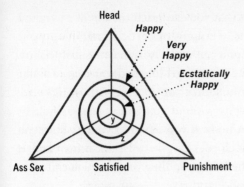

TOP VIEW

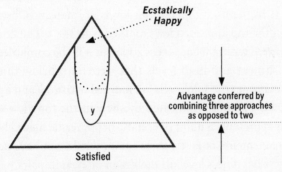

CENTER CUTAWAY

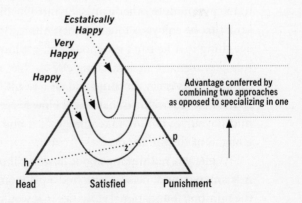

SIDE VIEW

A child understands that you can reach the top of a pyramid by climbing up one spine. Similarly, by participating in only one of these three activities, you can make Adrian ecstatically happy. For example, if every time you two get into bed you suck cock like his pre-cum is your only source for an essential amino acid, Adrian will be super-happy without going near your asshole or slapping any part of your body. If you sign over your asshole, you won't have to suck so much cock or take any punishment and, if he can spend as long as he wants paddling your ass, you can place your butthole out of service and reserve your mouth for special occasions.

If you don't want to specialize, you can offer a combination of two or three items at much lower levels of intensity. Observe the point on the top and side views marked with the z. The final position lies well within a happiness zone but it is the combined result of punishment and head levels that were both below the lowest happiness zone (the solo levels are marked with an h and a p in the side view). The point indicated by the y in the top view and the cutaway represents a point of ecstatic happiness achieved by using all three elements at levels that, again, would not have achieved the lowest happiness level on their own or even in pairs.

In addition to strategically combining Adrian's known areas of preference, you could change the game by adding another side to the pyramid: in other words, by introducing Adrian to a bit of kink that he enjoys as much as these three. Bring up some bondage thing that he can't get enough of, get him hooked on a sexy role-play scenario or something else . . . like maybe you grew up milking cows every morning and, as a result, you give a handjob so nuanced and refined that it will blow his mind. Adrian's pyramid is your pyramid. Take charge of it and decide how you're going to make him happy.

While you're thinking about how you'll position yourself on Adrian's pyramid, help Adrian find a place on yours. First, define the minimal foundational activities that would make your sex life satisfying. Then write the three or four corners of your own pyramid. If he's lucky, having your pussy eaten is one of them because you know he'll be going down on you like your lady juices are the antidote to a poison he's just ingested. It's kind of cheating, by the way, to pile everything you like into the foundation. (The person you cheat with this strategy is yourself.) Take the time it deserves to find the one, two, or three things you'd absolutely need to be satisfied in bed with him and put the rest into the pyramid.

YOUR FOUNDATION:

1. _____
2. _____
3. _____

YOUR PYRAMID CORNERS:

1. _____
2. _____
3. _____
4. _____

The Look

Not every experiment Adrian Colesberry tries will be a winner.[2] But for the health of your lovemaking, it's critical that you encourage his efforts. Easily done: Whenever he tries anything, like a new position, look at him like he's just executed the world's most difficult ice-skating maneuver. (This is especially important when things are not working out well.) Practice this look in the mirror. It should say, "Why, how did you come up with this magical configuration? My body would happily remain in this contortion for hours." Then, if it's uncomfortable, move immediately. Adrian isn't committed to the position itself, he just doesn't want to feel like an idiot inside that awkward moment of experimentation.

Experimenting

Once you've established a sexual routine that makes you both happy, it's still essential that you maintain an environment of change and experimentation. The shy reader may be thinking, "I don't have the moxie or brass or guts to experiment." That kind of fear is understandable, but what if you were told that Adrian Colesberry would be drawing out all your fantasies and desires in no time?

How, you wonder? Because Adrian understands that it's his job to be the pervert.[3]

According to what you've read so far, Adrian doesn't exactly need to encourage himself in that department, being plenty enough of a pervert without giving himself the job title. But here's the advantage you get from Adrian's conscious and triumphal perversion: He will never force you to be the pervert, even if it's something you've introduced. Say you finally get the guts up to ask him to fuck you in front of a mirror. Well, after that first time, he'll be the one to suggest that you fuck in front of the mirror. You won't have to put your neck out for it again. He's nothing if not a gentleman.

By faithfully following this ethic, Adrian will become the impossibly indebted pervert. His debt will demand the creation of more debt. His perversion will become the most valued commodity on the market. His debt will give you enough credit to be whoever you want to be, to demand whatever you want from him, to love him as openly and wildly as you can.

But even though he's shouldering your load in the pervert department, Adrian will not turn into a twentieth-century colonial power—assuming control over any part of your body you allow him to touch or imperialistically taking anything you bring up for experimental purposes and adding it to a list of things he has a right do to you from then forward. As a result of these policies, you can experiment in perfect freedom.[4]

Negotiation

Despite both of your good intentions, you may on rare occasions find yourself with a different sexual goal from that of Adrian Colesberry. You want to do something but he's reluctant, or he wants to do something and you're reluctant. Handled improperly, this situation can quickly and tragically lead to sexual gridlock, where both parties find that the only sexual freedom they can exercise is to deny the other person. Another equally tragic option is for one person to give in all the time. Neither of these options is acceptable, but Adrian's instinct told him that they were both avoidable.

In his bed, Adrian feels that he has the right to demand and the right to decline certain things and he feels that you also have the right to demand and the right to decline certain things. So he challenged himself to find a scientific way of determining the exact boundary between your rights and his.[5]

The System

Any sex act can be ranked on how much Adrian likes it or dislikes it physically and mentally, and the same applies to you. By averaging your results, a combined ranking can be generated for you as a couple, and this ranking will determine the right to demand or decline.

The system is represented by a grid. If your average falls in the upper-right quadrant, you'd do it without question. If in the lower-left quadrant, you wouldn't do it. If in the upper-left quadrant, the one with the desire has the right to demand; if in the lower-right quadrant, the one with the lack of desire has the right to decline.

It's that simple.

NEGOTIATION CHART

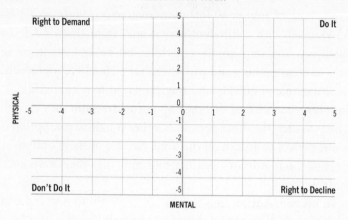

Fucking

There'd be no reason to develop a system if it was just for fucking. But to prove that the system can confirm a known fact: On a scale where –5 is the most disgusting and +5 the most exciting mental stimulation and where –5 is the most painful and +5 the most pleasurable physical stimulation, here is fucking for both Adrian and some fictional woman. Please put your own ranking in the blank box, calculate your average with Adrian, and plot your own point on the graph.

KEY TO THE NEGOTIATION CHARTS

♦   ■   ▲

ADRIAN   FICTIONAL WOMAN   FICTIONAL WOMAN & ADRIAN COMBINED

	◆ ADRIAN	■ FICTIONAL WOMAN	▲ FW & A COMBINED	YOU	You & A Combined
Physical	5	4	4.5		
Mental	4	4	4		

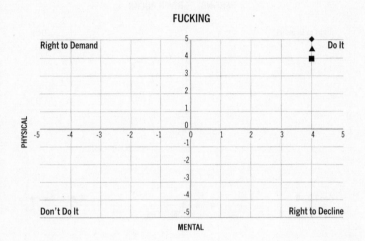

Since both ratings land in the upper-right, Do-It quadrant, it's no surprise that the combined rating, which is the midpoint of a line drawn between their individual ratings, lands in that quadrant too.

Pelting Each Other in the Head with Apple-Sized River Rocks

Again there's no reason to develop a system for things like this. No couple in their right minds would throw river rocks at each other—it's mutually physically painful and not a common fetish. Predictably, the chart plays out with each individual and also the combined scores landing in the Don't-Do-It quadrant. It's worrisome if you come up with a different result.

	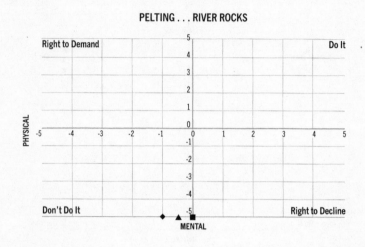 ADRIAN	FICTIONAL WOMAN	FW & A COMBINED	YOU	You & A Combined
Physical	-5	-5	-5		
Mental	-1	0	-0.5		

PELTING . . . RIVER ROCKS

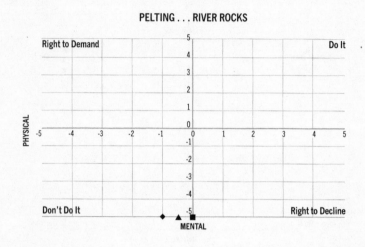

Head

Oral sex can be a point of conflict in relationships—not for Adrian, as you know, but just to test the system, pretend that he thinks giving head is disgusting. Adrian is rated below as a hypothetically reluctant cunniliguist, and the fictional woman as someone who quite naturally likes to get some head.

	ADRIAN, RELUCTANT PUSSY-EATER	FICTIONAL WOMAN	FW & A COMBINED	YOU	You & A Combined
Physical	0	4	2		
Mental	-3	4	.5		

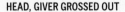

HEAD, GIVER GROSSED OUT

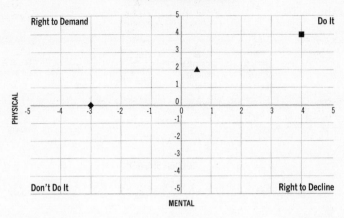

Giving head can't hurt unless you're doing it wrong, so the physical gets a score of zero. Observe that even though in this hypothetical eating pussy is somewhat mentally distressing to Adrian, the combined score falls cleanly inside the Do-It quadrant. If the tables were turned and you were the reluctant cocksucker, the result would be the same.

Golden Shower

Adrian has never tried this, but use the charts to see whether he would or not. He would certainly pee on you if you asked him to. Peeing by itself provides a mild physical pleasure that would in no way be decreased by having some part of your body interrupting his stream.

But what if you asked to pee on him? Physically, it would be a little stinky and hot, but not too unpleasant overall. Pee is a nearly sterile fluid, and assuming that the game was confined to the shower, or somewhere he could rinse off right after, the physical isn't really too bad. Mentally, it ranks in the negative for

Adrian. The fictional woman is ranked as a mild golden shower enthusiast.

	ADRIAN, GETTING PEED ON ◆	FICTIONAL WOMAN, ENTHUSED ■	FW & A COMBINED ▲	YOU	You & A Combined
Physical	-1	2	.5		
Mental	-4	3	-.5		

GOLDEN SHOWER

A surprising result, perhaps, but yes, if golden showers are what you're into, he'll let you pee on him.

Most important, keep in mind that these charts are the beginning of a negotiation, not the end. A dot on a graph on a piece of paper doesn't provide an excuse to throw courtesy or common sympathy out the window. You will never hear from Adrian Colesberry a complaint on the order of, "What do you mean, you don't feel like giving me a blowjob? Do I need to pull out the negotiation graph?" Impossible.

1 The Expert took a unique approach to Adrian's sexual menu. Anything he did to her, she would do right back to him. Some things worked out just brilliantly in her tit-for-tat universe: She didn't let him eat her box for two minutes before bucking him off to suck his cock in return. And needless to say, face-slapping was easy to arrange. Without being asked, she happily wailed away at his cheeks while he fucked her harder and harder. This barter system of hers was working out so far.

When he spanked her, she spanked him right back, lick for lick. It didn't help his erection any, but fair enough, right? After a few strokes, her smacks really began to smart. He'd never been spanked but once by the Kind One, and that apparently had been half-hearted. On experiencing, at the Expert's hand, his first real spanking, he realized that he didn't have enough fat back there to enjoy it. And the Expert had less fat on her ass than he did. A body needs a little padding to enjoy a spanking. He pretty quickly took spanking off the menu.

Don't make the mistake of thinking that the tit-for-tat will work to dismantle every part of Adrian's sexual program. Your tying him up won't send him the message that you don't like him tying you up, and if you don't like it when he goes down on you, it's probably not the best strategy to suck his cock until he gets it through his thick skull to keep his face out of your box. You can try, though. Doesn't hurt to try.

2 The disbelieving reader might want some proof that Adrian Colesberry is capable of a failed experiment, so here it is: The second time he fell in bed with the Enthusiast, she wrapped her tits around his cock and jerked him off with her cleavage. She didn't make a career of it or anything. It's just something she threw in occasionally as a variation on the blowjob she was giving him. Adrian thought this was wonderful and it gave him an idea: The next time he went down on her, he'd do the same thing and tit-fuck her as a variation on his box licking.

This flipping back and forth between cunnilingus and tit-fucking isn't something you'll be treated to, because it turned out to be geographically unrealistic in the extreme: When you're giving him a blowjob, mere inches will separate his cock from your cleavage, so you'll easily be able to transition back and forth if you'd like. But while eating your pussy, his cock and your tits will be separated by around four feet.

Not having made this calculation yet, Adrian waited until he was going down on her again, picked a moment, lifted his face out of the Enthusiast's box, and crawled up her body into the standard tit-fucking position—legs straddling her torso, knees planted in her armpits. By the end of this clumsy position change, he realized that he wouldn't be switching back and forth and felt neglectful for leaving his work between her legs unfinished. He could have thrown it into reverse, only that felt like retreating, so there he sat, his erection sandwiched in her cleavage without the will to finish what he'd so heroically started. Adrian felt like an idiot. It was in this moment that the Enthusiast saved the day by giving him the Look: gazing at him like he'd just executed the world's most difficult ice-skating maneuver. (See sidebar, page 147.)

3 Adrian didn't realize that it was his job to be the pervert until he started playing with the Great One's asshole. She thought his giving her rimjobs was so nasty that she couldn't stop reflexively moving her hips away from him when he did it. He had to pin her thighs beneath his chest to get a good run at her.

But still she let him do it, and every time she did, it was a little gift from her to him. After a month, he was in her debt for a few dozen rimjobs' worth, whatever that worked out to. And as it happened, he learned exactly what that worked out to—a spanking. It was only *after* the Great One figured he was enough in her debt that she asked him to spank her.

At that moment, the principle of being the first pervert among equals must unwittingly have formed in his subconscious, because after that first time, she never again had to ask him to spank her. He took over as the initiator of all the spanking. So aside from what he owed her for the rimjobs, he owed her for all the spankings, too; and when he tied her up, he owed her for that, and on and on until his debt became so enormous that any little kinky thing she requested would have been a drop in the bucket.

Adrian was doing great on this score with the Kind One until he blew it one morning and had to start all over again. They'd done a lot of spanking and slapping the previous evening (this was before the paddle). Over breakfast, Adrian commented, "Wow, you really get off on that, don't you?!"

The Kind One demanded, "*You* like it too, right?!" by which she was really saying, "Tell me right now that you like it at least as much as I do, or I'll be too humiliated to ever play that game again."

Adrian furiously backpedaled. "Are you kidding?! I'm all about the spanking!" He pointed out that it was he who had put them on that path to begin with. She hadn't started slapping herself in the face. After a few minutes of his gushing, she accepted the sincerity of his enthusiasm and returned to her scrambled eggs.

The sensible reader might wonder why the Kind One got so defensive. "Adrian was prudently and courteously checking for her consent. If he started spanking me, I'd want him to make sure I liked it." Sure you would. But he already knew that the Kind One liked it. And while it seems that he was just courtesy checking . . . he was doing something trickier beneath the surface.

Under cover of securing her consent, Adrian was foisting off onto her all the dirtiness associated with the punishment game. When he said, "Wow, you really get off on that, don't you?!" what he really meant was, "You like the spanking so crazy much, it doesn't really matter whether I like it or not. So let's agree that I'm not a part-time sadist at all but a do-gooder who benevolently spanks you as an act of charity." Only the Kind One was far too clever for his trick. She refused to take all that responsibility. To play the spanking game, she needed Adrian to be an unstoppable spank-crazy maniac who was going to spank her whether she wanted to be spanked or not.

A couple of months after nearly screwing everything up, his consistently playing the committed pervert got him back to a proper level of debt and produced results. They were getting dressed one morning when she picked up her underwear off the floor, held them out to him and challenged, "Try these on." Thrilled that she had walked through the now-wide-open door, he immediately stepped into them.

He'd never worn women's underwear before. They don't build them with enough room for man-tackle, so they were pretty tight, but otherwise very comfy.

He walked over to the mirror. They were aqua-blue silk, cut high up on his hips with two lace triangles in front that made kind of a diamond shape out of his crotch. He turned around. They did make his ass look tight. But the Kind One couldn't stop laughing, so he took them off.

If you want Adrian to wear your panties, when he pulls them on for the first time, start trying to suck his cock through the silk. Do that and his wearing panties might become a new thing for you two. Start finger-fucking yourself while he models them and he might never wear any other kind.

4 The Wednesday after he'd introduced skull-fucking, they were lying on their sides 69ing when suddenly the Kind One flipped onto her back, pulled him on top, grabbed his ass, and had him fuck her mouth. Adrian was delighted that she was getting with the program so quickly.

A few strokes in, he noticed that he was pushing deeper than usual. After about a minute, she spit out his cock and started gasping for air. As soon as she could get the words out, she explained, "I forgot to breathe." She'd been letting him fuck her throat.

Adrian thought that her experience of airlessness would mark the end of her little experiment, but, on catching her breath, she started the cycle all over again. She'd undertaken the project of getting properly fucked in the throat and wasn't going to let one tiny glitch hinder its achievement. Not a quitter . . . Adrian respected that.

And here's the coolest thing. The Kind One never had him fuck her throat again, not ever. He watched to see if it would come up . . . but no. She'd tried it out. She hadn't liked it. She'd dropped it. Somehow, she realized that she could trust him to ride that ride with her, then trust him to get off the ride when she wanted off.

5 After fucking you for any period of time, Adrian will bring up the idea of getting you a vibrator. He even has a sales pitch to go with this suggestion: He'll say a word about how it would be great to have a vibrator when Adrian Colesberry isn't there to give you the attention you deserve. And when Adrian is in the neighborhood, it might be fun for him to fuck you with it or watch as you fucked yourself with it or for you to buzz your clitoris with it while he fucked you or for him to go down on you while fucking you with it . . . He figures that one of these things will sound like a good time.

You might greet his suggestion with, "Thanks, I've got one already. Want to see what I do with it?" (Yes, he would.) Or "I've never had a vibrator, but it sounds like fun, let's go get one." (Nice. He will go get you one.) Or "I don't have one, but I'd rather not." (OK. He'll ask again in two months.) What he wasn't expecting was the reply that came out of the Great One's mouth: "If we get one, you aren't going to try and put it up my ass, are you?"

Reader, please think of Adrian Colesberry more charitably than this. The woman had specifically told him she didn't even want his finger up her ass! What did she think he was thinking?! "So, no on my finger, no on my penis . . . I know what she wants up her ass! A cock-shaped slug of injection-molded rubber with imbedded electrical components."

Out loud, Adrian calmly insisted that he had no such plans for the vibrator and reminded her that they'd already agreed that nothing at all would go up her ass. She seemed reassured but he felt that the continued freedom of their lovemaking was in jeopardy.

He had to figure out some way to convince her, once and for all, that he didn't think she was being ungenerous by refusing him ass sex. But before he could convince her, he'd have to figure out why *he* didn't resent the Great One for not giving up her ass. More important, how do you know he won't resent you if you don't let him put his cock in your ass?

Ass sex would certainly be a good time as far as he's concerned. It's nasty. *Check.* It involves putting his penis into a warm hole. *Check.* He likes playing with your asshole in other ways. *Check.* So how does he not feel deprived when you keep his penis out of there? This intellectual and moral crisis was the crucible in which Adrian created his negotiation charts.

The charts he showed to the Great One clearly demonstrated her right to refuse a dildo up her ass.* They got that vibrator.

Inconveniently, the chart he worked up on ass-fucking landed in his Right-to-Demand quadrant. Needless to say, he didn't include that chart in his presentation to the Great One.

Love

Fidelity

Startup Fidelity

At the beginning of a relationship with Adrian, it's not sound policy to assume that he's dating only you, but at the same time it's a bit too early to talk about exclusivity. The pro tip is to postpone that conversation until you've gotten Adrian addicted to the pussy or at the very least given him a taste. He will greet a conversation about monogamy before you've slept together much the same way you'd greet a conversation about ass sex before he's taken you out to dinner.

If your self-esteem is crying out that you deserve a man who is completely focused on you, know that Adrian Colesberry firmly agrees that you deserve that. It's his penis that's the problem: It will not allow Adrian to place exclusivity before sex, and Adrian will have to wait for its approval before he makes you the one and only.

Exclusive Relationships

Once you and Adrian have agreed to be exclusive in your relationship, he will not fuck around on you. This isn't some lame promise, but a disinterested prediction drawn from the facts of his personal history. If you talked to him about his never being un-faithful, he might feel somehow obligated as a man to add, "Not that I didn't have the opportunity." (But he didn't.[1])

It's not like he's a moral hero. By being faithful he's just acting in protection of his own happiness. If he's constantly thinking about how he could be fucking other people, this would tragically transform him from being the guy who's fucking you to being the guy who's *not* fucking all those other people. It's a glass-half-full/glass-half-empty thing. Being the guy who's fucking you is pretty great. He can spend his time thinking about what he's going to do to you next and how you're so incredibly nasty for letting him do what he did to you the last time.

The Devil's in the Details

Aside from being a part of his character, there are a couple of technical reasons that Adrian won't fuck around on you. First, he's not the neatest person in the world. He can't keep up the cleaning schedule required to remove all the blond curly hairs from his bathroom and bedroom before the straight-haired bru-nette shows up. (Don't get the impression that Adrian's environ-ment is some kind of pigsty. He's just not all that tidy.)

The second and main reason he won't fuck around on you is that he's a terrible liar—world-class terrible. Keeping a surprise party secret for your birthday will drive him to distraction—and a surprise birthday party is a nice thing. There's no way he's ca-pable of telling the thousand little lies needed to keep a betrayal from you like, "You're sharing my cock with another lover or three."

But being the guy who isn't fucking all those other ladies . . . that's a horror show. Every woman who walks by represents a personal failure. He's an incurable loser by the end of the day and you're the consolation prize. (Lucky you.) Adrian can't live like that.

Open Relationships

Make no mistake, Adrian would love it if you were happy to share his cock with other ladies, in which case, he wouldn't make any monogamy demands on you, either. There are three basic ways this kind of thing works out: honest philandering, polyamory, and a fuck-buddy arrangement. A closer examination will reveal which, if any, would be possible for Adrian Colesberry.

1. Honest Philandering

Adrian announces to you early on, "I fuck other women. Get it? If you want to be with me, you need to be OK with that." This is not going to happen because Adrian doesn't have the off-the-charts self-esteem necessary to carry this out.

2. Polyamory

After a deep-into-the-night conversation about how human beings are all really one, spiritually speaking, and how love is this infinite, amazing force that no social institution could possibly put in a box, Adrian suggests that you could really stick it to culture and its strangulating boundaries by letting him share his love (cock) with everyone in the world (one or two other ladies he's had his eye on). Adrian couldn't get through the first part of that conversation without laughing and definitely wouldn't be able to pull off the second part. From his, perhaps spiritually unenlightened, perspective, this kind of arrangement too often involves one person who really wants to fuck around and another person who wants to be with the first person so much that they're willing to put up with it, and that seems to him a little sad.

3. Fuck Buddies

You and Adrian both find yourself in a place where you want to have a sexual relationship but neither of you wants the encumbrances of a boyfriend/girlfriend relationship. In general, Adrian is OK with this. He'll have to be sure that you're not just saying you'll be fuck buddies because you think it's the only way he'll be with you and you're betting that he'll get addicted to the pussy. That would make him sad again. Not to encourage this gamble, but he probably will get addicted to the pussy and, even though you've agreed that you're just fuck buddies, won't do much or any fooling around.[2]

Breaking Up

If he breaks up with you, Adrian will not tell you how horrible you are or criticize you in any way. Anyone overhearing the breakup would think that you were an angel visiting the earth from the wonderful things he'll say about you.[3]

Adrian will lie about why he wants out. In his mind, he does this to preserve your feelings. It will not preserve your feelings. It will make you more confused and upset. It will, however, preserve Adrian's feelings because in that moment the real reason he is breaking up with you, regardless of how much sense it makes, will seem to him like the most heartless, horrible thing in the world.

If he was moving to a different continent, Adrian would tell you that he found someone else just so you wouldn't think your decision not to move with him was the cause of the breakup. And if he'd found someone else, he just might tell you that he was moving to a different continent, so you wouldn't be hurt by his absented affections.

Adrian will not cry, unless you show any emotion. If you show any emotion at all, he will cry like a baby. Just as he is not equipped for make-up sex, he is also not equipped for breakup sex. So get that one final romp right out of your head.[4]

Adrian ends relationships quickly. It'll be over in a day—less than that if you're the one breaking up with Adrian. That's the easiest. Once you tell Adrian you don't want to see him any longer, he's out. He won't make a single argument. He can't stand the idea of spending a second with someone who doesn't want to spend time with him. Breaking up with Adrian is kind of like an ancient nomadic divorce ritual where the woman turns her tent to face the opposite direction and the next time her man returns to camp he finds out that he's divorced. No fuss.[5]

I Love You

If Adrian Colesberry is fucking you, he is loving you. That's what "I love you" means as far as Adrian is concerned, and he deeply wishes he would have had the guts to spend his whole life saying it when he felt it.[6] But unfortunately, Adrian has fallen sway to the social prejudice that forbids you to express love the way you do other emotions—say, happiness.

If Adrian said to you, "I'm happy," you wouldn't think that he was swearing to be happy only around you or promising to be happy all the time. People who are happy all the time get tossed into insane asylums. Life is not a happy-all-the-time proposition. But for some reason, if he says "I love you," that means "I love you now and that feeling is never going to change or be transferred to anybody else . . . ever."

This form of "I love you" has only appeared in his longest-term relationships. But the longer these relationships lasted, the more "I love you" came to mean "Good-bye" or "I've got to go." If pronounced emphatically, it meant, "Seriously, my boss is standing in my cubicle like two feet away from me. I have *got* to *go!*"[7]

The careful reader won't want to dilute Adrian's "I love you" to the point that it means "Even though I'm hanging up the phone,

I don't hate you." If you do, by definition, Adrian loves everyone just as much as he loves you, except for a handful of telemarketers (the rude ones, not the nice ones).

Here are the only times when you should expect (or want) Adrian to say that he loves you:

- He wants to fuck you.
- You're fucking him at the moment.
- You've just finished fucking him.
- It's a special moment that doesn't necessarily have to have anything to do with fucking (these do exist for Adrian Colesberry).
- You're about to be separated for a while.
- You need emotional reinforcement, and he's accurately assessed that you'd like to hear that he loves you.
- Adrian himself needs emotional reinforcement.
- Nothing in particular is going on, but he's blindsided by the fact that he loves you.

Beyond these situations, make sure he keeps it in his pocket.

If the relationship goes on for long enough, your "I love you" will inevitably become commonplace. But all is not lost. You just have to come up with another way to say the "I love you" that means "I can't get enough of you right now. Where did you come from? How could I deserve you?" It doesn't even need to be words; it could be a hand gesture—anything.

Love vs. Fucking

From all this less-than-lofty talk about love, you might be getting the mistaken notion that Adrian is a mighty cynic on the subject. Not at all. Adrian is very much a romantic. Only, as far as love goes, he's also very much an agnostic. He doesn't believe in it; he doesn't *not* believe in it; he just doesn't want to talk about it. If you love him, he wants to experience the evidence of those feelings and he'll give you evidence of his love in return.

This is where Adrian finds fucking to be so fantastic. Your feeling that you want to fuck Adrian Colesberry is nice, just like your feeling that you love him is nice. But there's no amount of energy that Adrian can expend to fuck himself *for* you. You can say, "I fuck you" all day long, but by the end of the night, either you've fucked him or you haven't fucked him.

That's why Adrian will establish up-front a lovemaking that is lengthy and involved: He needs to know the truth about whether you want him or not, and he can only judge your interest in fucking him if he can fuck for long enough to truly put your interest to the test. Leaving him with the following problem: How can he make sure that he can fuck you for long enough? Don't spend your time thinking about this question, because Adrian has already come up with an answer—actually three: exercise, napping, and snacking.

At the gym, Adrian directly addresses the physical limitations that he's encountered during your last time in bed together (abdominals, endurance, lower back, whatever) so that he can fuck you for longer the next time.[8] And if he gets tired while you're fucking, he'll take a nap.[9] And if he needs to recharge his energy, he'll have a snack.[10]

So when Adrian falls asleep, understand that it's not over. Even when he finally knocks off for the evening, he's really just resting so he can fuck you better in the morning. And it's not just the snacks he eats while you're fucking, but every meal on days that you're getting together and also on days you're apart. And it's not just the sleeping and the food: At the gym, he's staying in shape so he can fuck you. At the movies, he's culturally recharging so he can fuck you. At work he's making money so he can fuck you. In an important and very real way, Adrian is fucking you all the time.

He'll fuck you and nap and fuck you some more and snack and fuck you even more and work out and fuck you again until there is no possible question that a lot, meaning *a lot*, of fucking has gone on, because no one in their right mind (especially not someone as mentally well balanced as you) would put up with that much fucking if you did not really, *really,* want him to be fucking you.[11]

At some point, if you are not *completely* into fucking him you'll say, "Uncle!" or "I'm tired" or "Please just stop" or "Let's go to sleep if you can't cum" or "Get off me" or something. And while you might put up with all that business one or two times, there's no possible way that you'll come back for the twentieth round of his fucking you and napping and snacking and then waking you up—if you decide to nap also, which he will encourage—and fucking you some more if you don't truly and for sure want him. There is force of logic behind his way of thinking.

Is Adrian Thinking About How He Loves Me?

When you look at Adrian in the act, you may wonder what's going through his head. Easily answered. In his unfocused moments, he's mostly thinking about an errand he has to run or whether the chicken that he bought a few days ago is still good or whether he'll have to throw it out or another fragment of the pointless miscellany that orbits around his brain. But in those moments where you'd be most likely to wonder what in the world is summoning that look of intensity and love, Adrian is thinking about how you are a collection of holes that he can fuck (or fill with his fingers or a toy or something or other).

If that disturbs you and you think it would be nice for Adrian to take a break from violating you in his mind and at least occasionally think about how he loves you or how you're darling, you're wrong. It wouldn't be nice. It would be a waste of time.

Your mistake is in thinking that love is an emotion. It's not. Love is an action, or a collection of actions. It's all the things Adrian has done for you and his promise to keep doing those things in the future. While he's fucking you, the action that Adrian can take to love you in that moment is to fuck you properly. And he is most able to do that when he thinks about how you are a collection of holes he can fuck.

You must know that he does think you're darling. And he has as many sentimental and soft thoughts as you'd like. He thinks those thoughts all the time, like when he's cooking you dinner or when he's keeping his mouth shut during an argument where you're just crabby and are saying a bunch of things you're going to feel sorry for in a few minutes. His soft thoughts help him then; they just don't help him in bed.

He doesn't put his tongue up your asshole because he loves you or wants you to have his babies or hopes to grow old with you and sit out the long afternoons on a porch swing feeling the same breeze cool off your two bodies. Adrian puts his tongue up your asshole or gets it up to fuck you again after only a few minutes' break or figures out something new to do with your clitoris because he thinks of you as a collection of holes that he can fuck.

Take some time to think it through and you'll realize that you wouldn't want it any other way.

CHAPTER 9 NOTES

1 The closest Adrian ever came to fucking around on the Wife was when a friend of hers moved into their apartment building. Only days after he heaved the friend's sofa against the wall of an apartment two floors down, the Wife's behavior toward her formerly close companion turned rude and mean. When he asked what the deal was, she pointed out how her friend full-on flirted with him every time she came over. He hadn't noticed, but now that she'd mentioned it, he started to. Flattering!

Unfortunately, all the friend's flirting made the Wife even more unpleasant to live with, and the fact that this woman would flirt with her friend's husband made her a bit creepy. Plus, his own wife had pimped her out to him. He couldn't hit that! What's the rap for that situation? "Hey. Your friend, you know, my wife, said that you might want to fuck me?"

Like most women, the Wife no doubt had a hundred opportunities better than this one. But she probably didn't fuck around on him either. Nothing to her credit. She didn't like sex that much in the first place. Counting her fidelity as a virtue would be like congratulating an anorexic on holding back at an all-you-can-eat buffet.

Once-bitten reader, despite these reassurances that Adrian is not susceptible to infidelity, you may still want to know if there are any indications that he is thinking about it. There is one sign: reverse jealousy.

Throughout their marriage, the Wife would say and do little things intended to make him jealous, like point out when men were looking at her or flirting with her, even when they weren't. If a jealous man is what really turns you on, Adrian will do his best to oblige, but he's not very jealous by nature and it's absolutely impossible to make him jealous if you're not fucking him like the Wife wasn't.

For a couple of years before the end, when she pulled her little stunt, he'd not only fail to see the man as a rival but would see him as a savior who might take this albatross from around his neck, so he'd push her to go chat up the offending store clerk, bar patron, or museumgoer. If Adrian starts encouraging you, however subtly, to fuck around on him, that's a bad sign.

2   Despite his stellar potential as a fuck buddy, Adrian's first-ever open relationship didn't materialize until a year after his divorce, when he met the Kind One at a Wednesday-night pottery class taught by a locally famous, master ceramicist. After their last class, they went out for dinner to say good-bye. As the plates were cleared, he could have offered to stay friends, but the Kind One didn't want a friend. She wanted something else. She'd spent most of the meal talking about how, in her marriage (also recently dissolved), the sex had deteriorated to the point where she basically hadn't gotten laid for five years. He knew how that felt and told her so. Trying to be helpful, Adrian encouraged her to jump back on that horse. Dating isn't as intimidating as it seems, and all that business.

The Kind One kept looking at him like he'd spilled gravy on his shirt until he finally got the hint that she didn't want his advice for the newly single. She wanted Adrian Colesberry. Not as a boyfriend or anything. She'd made it very clear that she wouldn't have any part of that.

The Kind One needed a friend to help her back onto that horse, so Adrian immediately threw the idea of being fuck buddies onto the table. If you want to be fuck buddies with Adrian Coles-berry, don't worry that you will have to come out and say it. He's aware that your suggesting it might make you seem a little desperate, whereas he, a man, Adrian Colesberry, could print up business cards with his picture on it and the question, "Do you want to be fuck buddies?" and hand them out to every woman he met without seeming desperate in any way.

Once the relationship had been officially declared, they established the rules of engagement, mainly worked out by the Kind One, who had apparently come to their last class with a plan. In principle, fuck-buddy rules are meant to nip in the bud those normal expectations that sprout up in normal relationships. Your exact rules could be different of course, but this template shows what bases you need to cover.

RESTRICTION	THE KIND ONE'S RULE	DISCUSSION
Where you will meet	He would not come to her house; she would come to his. That would be their place.	The Kind One was being particularly stringent here. You can go to both of your houses or even include a restaurant among the meeting places, but the possible locations should be defined.
What you will do	There would be no dating. He would be no boyfriend. There would only be the sex.	This could be expanded to include eating a meal beforehand. It could also be far narrower, allowing only certain acts.
When you will meet	Wednesday. That would be their day.	The time restriction is probably the most important. Even if it is not a single day, it should be limited somehow: weekdays only, weekends only. But the designated weekday is the classic choice.

These restrictions were important to the Kind One because her past boyfriends and ex-husband had misconstrued her inviting them into her vagina as an invitation to become the boss of her life besides. She very much wanted to invite Adrian into her vagina, but didn't want him spoiling things by getting all bossy.

Whether in a fuck-buddy relationship or not, those fears are unwarranted with Adrian Colesberry. He has enough on his hands making his own life decisions and has no desire to make yours for you. Lending Adrian your vagina, along with whatever other parts you'll throw into the deal, will never involve any compromise to your free will.

Though he saw the strictness of the Kind One's rules as unnecessary, Adrian was OK with them. His penis worked better at his house anyway, and if he wanted to go see a movie, he could go with a buddy he wasn't fucking and, for months, he had kept Wednesday nights clear for the ceramics class so it would be easy to continue keeping it for this new purpose. And he only saw the Great One on the weekends, so it didn't interfere with that. To seal the deal, they kissed on the sidewalk by her car. It was a good kiss. It was a great kiss. This was going to work out just fine.

3 Naturally enough, the First One was the first woman Adrian ever broke up with. For weeks, he'd wanted to end it, but couldn't figure out how. Then the school year ended, and he just didn't tell her where he was moving to. It was cowardly and cruel. Even worse, it didn't work. Somehow, she got ahold of his new number and called to ask if they could fuck one last time.

He gave in, of course. They met up, kissed for a minute, she humped his leg for two minutes until she came, she sucked his cock for one minute, and then he fucked her for two minutes until he came. Just like old times. Then they got dressed and went their separate ways and he thought that was that. But two months later, she called again. She told him that in an unsuccessful attempt to get pregnant, she'd stopped taking the Pill the day after their last get-together. Adrian wasn't yet bright enough to protect himself by wearing a condom.

After the First One, it was a while before he had to break up with anybody . . . but then he had to break up with everybody.

The summer after his junior year, he met the Wife (who wasn't yet his wife) at a big ceramics university where he'd gone for a study program. When he got back in town, he started the process of closing down all his college relationships. On this round of breakups, he made one improvement in strategy—he didn't tell anyone that they were breaking up and then go off and fuck them one last time. (That whole incident with the First One can explain why he's incapable of breakup sex.)

The Deliberate One was easy. He didn't really have to break up with her at all. She'd gone back to her boyfriend, never having gotten out of Adrian the one strange fuck that she wanted. The Talker was pretty painless too. She'd heard about the Wife from a mutual friend and stopped coming around.

The Loved One, Adrian dealt with properly. He called her a couple of days after he got back into town and asked her to dinner. As soon as he walked into her dorm room to pick her up, she guessed, "You're breaking up with me."

She said she'd known it since before he left but, hedging against her own premonition, had starved herself all summer to make her ass smaller for him. There's no telling where she got the idea that Adrian wanted her ass to be smaller. He'd only ever thought that she had a perfect ripe peach of an ass.

Saying that she wanted him to at least inspect the results of her hard work, she emerged from the bathroom naked and paraded around. He agreed that it looked smaller, declining to mention that it looked no better, not to him at least. Afterward, she put on her clothes and let him take her out to dinner, then he broke up with her like he'd planned.

Two days later, the Loved One called to tell him that she hadn't had her period since before he left town. The contraceptive-aware reader might be shocked that Adrian would find himself in this position again, but before you jump to conclusions, Adrian had learned his lesson from the First One. He had never fucked the Loved One without a condom.

They met again for dinner and he asked her if she had a plan. Well yes, she did: She planned to drop out of college, have the baby, and raise it on her grandmother's farm. You can imagine his relief. He was ready to freak out if she hadn't had a plan, but as long as she was willing to completely arrest the forward progress of her life and hide away on a farm until the baby was born and possibly stay there for the rest of her life . . . He started crying right in the middle of the restaurant.

Regardless of his strong feelings, Adrian didn't try to talk her into an abortion. In his mind, he'd given over his reproductive control the second he ejaculated. All he said was, "I'll help out any way I can." Like maybe he could drive her to the family farm so Grandma could meet the dirty, dirty boy who had polluted her precious granddaughter with his vile seed.

When the Loved One went to the doctor and got tested, it turned out that she wasn't pregnant after all; she'd just stifled her ovulation that summer by smoking pot nonstop and starving herself to make her ass smaller.

4 The most-improved feature of his postdivorce breakups over his pre-divorce breakups is the lack of any pregnancy scares. The Enthusiast and Adrian just stopped calling each other by tacit, mutual agreement. The Innocent One wanted a boyfriend, and since Adrian wasn't going to be her boyfriend, she decided that she didn't want to fuck him anymore. Fair enough.

His breakup with the Great One was complicated by the fact that neither of them wanted it to happen. One weekend, in a series of incredibly stupid moves, Adrian revealed to her that he was still interested in seeing other women. Following protocol, he lied about the exact form his interest was taking: He said he was dating around on her but didn't mention that he was fucking around on her.

In fact, he wasn't doing any dating, but for a month he had been fuck buddies with the Kind One. It probably would have hurt the Great One less to hear the truth—while he was entirely uninterested in serious dating, he needed a fuck exactly midweek to hold him over. But that's how Adrian breaks up.

On hearing he was still dating, the Great One was devastated. He was devastated that she was devastated. He tried not to cry and ended up crying more than he would have if he'd just let himself cry in the first place. She asked if they could fuck one last time. He said he couldn't. He admitted that they had not had the I'm-dating-other-people conversation. She admitted that they had not had the I'm-not-dating-other-people conversation. They broke up that same day. They'd never even had one fight, but they didn't have a choice—he couldn't ask her to tolerate his fucking around and she couldn't ask him to commit.

Adrian was in love with the Great One. He stayed in love with her for a long time. But as he'd learned in his marriage, loving someone, really loving someone, isn't what you feel toward that person but what you are willing to do for that person. So regardless of how much Adrian felt that he loved the Great One, he obviously didn't love her enough.

Adrian does not anticipate ever breaking up with you, but just in case, take some pictures because if he ever has to go through the process of missing you, he'd like a picture to miss you with. Adrian sure wished he'd had a picture of the Great One. He was shocked that they could have loved so freely, yet left their lives together unrecorded. He felt disoriented, like she'd been a fit of his imagination. In the absence of photographs, he collected all the evidence he could find that she had existed at all.

The Hair. He gathered a few pieces and made a tangle of it.

The Hickey. The last time they made love, she gave him a hickey on his bicep. If he pushed it, it still hurt. He photographed it every day until it faded away. Now at least, he had some pictures.

The Cuff. As they were breaking up on her couch, she kept fidgeting with the sleeve of his leather jacket. A few days later, he noticed that his cuff was still turned up in the position where she'd folded it. He decided to leave it that way. It could fall back into place naturally, but he would not himself undo her work.

Weeks after the hickey had disappeared, the cuff was still there. Then one day, he was reaching into the dairy case at his grocery store to grab a carton of cottage cheese when a perfect stranger bumped his arm. She excused herself, then, thinking that their collision had somehow folded his sleeve into the Great One's sloppy cuff, she did the motherly thing and turned it back down.

And that was the very end.

5   The exception to the short breakup was his marriage, which took him anywhere from two to ten years to end, depending on when you start the clock. About two years before the end, he gave up on hoping that the Wife's freelance career would go places or that she would in any way turn into a competent partner and started insisting that she get a job, any job, so that she could at least give him a break from being the only breadwinner.

After seriously considering his request, the Wife counterproposed that Adrian could get an even better break by having a mental-health professional declare him unfit to perform his work at the factory due to psychological stress and then going on disability leave at two-thirds pay for the rest of his productive life. Always the team player, Adrian agreed to pursue a career in mental disability with the understanding that she would pursue a career period.

At his first therapy session, Adrian started out complaining exclusively about his job at the factory, as they'd planned, but the therapist asked about his family and his marriage and he ended up telling her as much of his life story as he could push out. After fifty minutes, she concluded that his problems came from his marriage, which wasn't giving him one single thing that he needed, including sex.

The Wife was furious when he came home without a certificate of insanity and thought he was being plainly perverse when he decided to go back and talk to the same lady for a second session instead of moving on through the insurance list until he found a health professional with enough vision to see that his job, and his job alone, was pushing him to the verge of a mental meltdown.

Flash forward to a year and a half later and, one day, Adrian, sitting in his office at work, caught himself thinking about which women in his social circle would fuck him even though they knew he was married. Everybody daydreams about fucking other people, but this wasn't a daydream. He was compiling a list. Not a jerk-off list. An action list. A list of specific women in the exact order that he would approach them.

When he snapped out of his list-making, what he'd been doing hit him like a ton of bricks. That guy who fucks around on his wife in a deliberate, strategic way . . . that guy wasn't him. He was turning into someone he didn't even recognize.

He picked up the phone and called the Wife to tell her how unhappy he was. As soon as she heard his voice, she guessed, "You're leaving me, aren't you?" She knew how much of a coward he was about saying the hard things, so she said the hard thing for him. She could be sweet sometimes.

In the remote possibility that Adrian wants to break up with you, it would be great if you could catch on to what he's doing and kind of break up with yourself for him. Say whatever you'd like to hear. "It's not me; it's you." He'll agree with everything you say and try not to cry. Then he'll cry anyway.

6 The Loved One, from back in college, was the first person outside his family to say that she loved him. He was right up inside her and she just blurted it out. He must have tensed up, because she immediately backpedaled. "I just want to say that. Do you mind? You don't have to say it back. But can I still say it?"

Well of course she could. That's a "Can I sit here?" kind of question. Unless someone is actually sitting there, you say yes. And since no one else was lining up to tell him they loved him, sure, she could go ahead and say it. So after that, every time they had sex, during her second orgasm, the one she had while fucking, not the one she had in his mouth, she told him she loved him.

He felt plain mean not saying it back. It's not that he didn't feel it . . . he *did* love her for fucking him and for wanting him so much. He loved her for telling him that she loved him. If he didn't love her, why else did he love fucking her so much?

But at the time, he was sleeping with the Deliberate One and the Talker, so it felt like a lie somehow. He felt that if he loved her enough, he wouldn't need two other women to service his sex drive, so he never said it even though he felt it so strongly.

The low-self-esteem reader might be thinking, "Yeah, but that was the Loved One. Adrian would never feel so strongly about me, much less say it out loud." So not true. What the Loved One noticed was that while fucking Adrian Colesberry, she was already loving him, so in a way saying "I love you" out loud didn't add any new information.

7   The Wife ended up being the first person to hear from Adrian the kind of "I love you" that means "I love you and this feeling is never going to change, ever." He heard it from her a lot, so to avoid building up an "I love you" deficit, every time she said it, he'd fire back with, "I love you too." But it turned out that no amount of "I love you too" or "back atcha" or "ditto" or pointing his finger back at her in a funny way counted against the deficit. The only "I love you" that counted was an originally stated "I love you." So he got in the habit of saying, "I love you" to her a lot . . . a lot, a lot, a lot.

At first, when he said it, he meant that he loved her and that his feelings would not change, but over the years his "I love you" took on different meanings, most of them having nothing to do with love.

The Wife arranged her life so that she had a ton of spare time, meaning she had no job. Whenever she got bored, which was often, she'd call him up at his work and talk his ear off, but he couldn't listen to her all day since people were paying him to do stuff that had nothing to do with talking to her.

She would only stop talking when he hung up, but if he just banged the phone down, she'd call right back all upset that he'd hung up on her and waste even more of his workday, so he got in the habit of saying "I love you," then hanging up right after. She wouldn't get mad if the last thing she'd heard out of his mouth was an "I love you."

Attentive reader, Adrian's substituting "I love you" for "good-bye" is a very bad sign. He only does it when he thinks your mental health requires constant reinforcement of his affection and a constant restatement of his promise to stick around in your life. You do not want Adrian thinking about you in this way. The less and less Adrian loved the Wife, the more and more she needed to hear that he loved her. He obliged, but quantity is, as in all things, not quality.

Once "I love you" and "good-bye" had become synonyms, Adrian started to ring off with coworkers by telling them that he loved them. If he caught himself in time, he'd tag "man" on the end to make it "I love you . . . man!" Then he'd laugh like he'd just made a super-great joke.

Once though, he told the vice president of Human Resources that he loved him but he couldn't man-tag it because he didn't catch himself until after hanging up. Adrian called right back and asked him, "Did I just tell you that I loved you?" He had. How awkward.

In a corporate environment, you don't casually break up with an executive officer, especially not immediately after announcing the relationship, so Adrian didn't feel like he could explain, "Sorry. I *don't* love you. That's just what I say sometimes when I really have to get off the phone."

And no need, because the man didn't leave him hanging for a second. He said, "I love you too, Adrian." Those are some gigantic people skills. No wonder he was the vice president of Human Resources.

8 Adrian's stomach muscles will be the first to go. When fucking in missionary, he holds himself in what a yoga teacher might call the half-cobra position—his arms locked at the elbow, holding his torso up off his body. As he found out with the Great One, in this position his stomach muscles drive his hip movements. Toward Sunday evening, his abdomen would start seizing up midthrust. He was already doing 180 crunches three times a week, so to solve the problem he upped his crunches to 240 and added 60 leg raises.

The weekend after this exercise change, his stomach held up like a trooper. But Monday morning, he woke up with painful, knotty cramps in each buttock. To correct this, he began doing reverse lunges. For each leg, he did two sets of ten repetitions with 50 pounds on the bar. After two weeks of reverse lunges, his buttocks stopped cramping up.

Next, his wrists will start hurting from bearing all his weight. For this, he'll do wrist curls. After that, his lower back will seize up, so he needs to stretch out more and increase from two to three sets his lower back crunches, where he lies on his stomach and does reverse sit-ups. After that, he'll begin to ache in his inner thigh and groin, which he can solve using that leg-squeeze machine at the gym.

Once he's solved all his skeletal muscle failures, one last problem will crop up—his heart. With the Great One, he couldn't fuck fast for more than a couple of minutes without getting coronary-arrest-style chest pains. After some experimentation, he started using the stair stepper to do a series of short wind sprints, which mimics how he has sex anyway—fuck and stop, fuck and stop.

9 With the Kind One Adrian discovered another way to make sex last, when one evening he caught himself dropping off to sleep while eating her out. The third time that he picked his face up out of her snatch, she looked down at him and suggested, "Why don't we take a nap."

His first impulse was to say, "I'm fucking! Not sleeping!" But he's sensitive to the needs of other people and if *she* was tired, he was happy to keep her company. He passed out as soon as his head hit the pillow. She was reading a book when he woke up, rested and erect, an hour later. From then on, whenever he got tired, he'd take a nap then wake up fresh for more fucking.

10 Even with a lot of napping, Adrian still found himself running out of steam. Then one night, after the Kind One went to the bathroom, he got up to clean the kitchen and just as he was scraping her half-eaten dinner into the trash, he realized that he was starving, so he scraped it into his mouth instead. He called out to her. "I just ate the rest of your food. I hope you were finished." She said she was, but he still wasn't, so he made himself a half of a peanut butter and marmalade sandwich. Then he took his nap.

She emerged from the bathroom, expecting to fall asleep on his shoulder. But he woke up and started fucking her instead. From then on, they structured all their fucking like infant day care—with regular snack breaks and nap times for Baby Adrian.

11 There was one exception to the rule of lengthy lovemaking: Save for that first night when it took his penis a while to come online, Adrian and the Expert never fucked for more than five minutes at a stretch.

Their typical sexual exchange boiled down to a minute of oral sex each way, a couple of minutes fucking her snatch and a couple of minutes fucking her ass. Adrian would barely have established a rhythm before she'd urgently push him off, roll on her side and, while holding onto his erection with one hand, masturbate herself with the other or with a bullet vibrator she had. She'd encourage him to jerk off on her tits after she'd cum, but there was no way he was ready to do that after only five minutes, so they'd go out for a drink or a bite or just watch TV until she was ready to fuck again—for five more minutes.

The sympathetic reader can imagine how much this distressed Adrian. The only reason he kept coming around was because the Expert packed those five minutes of fucking with incredibly high levels of kink. But all that short-attention-span sex ended once she started finger-banging his asshole. If he wanted to get his cock sucked for fifteen minutes instead of the usual two, all he had to do was flip her into a position where she could reach his asshole and: done—like putting a quarter in a parking meter.

What is your version of finger-banging Adrian Colesberry in the ass? Maybe, like the Kind One, it's getting a spanking. That would be good news. Maybe it's having him eat your snatch? More good news. Or maybe it's something totally random, like you want to be filmed. Ten minutes is good enough with no photo documentation, but with the camera rolling, you can be fucked for hours. Sounds like fun, actually. Adrian's never filmed anything so will definitely sign up for that.

Sex Talk

Be aware that Adrian will be reporting to at least one close friend the minutest details of your body and your sexual encounters—which of your boobs hangs lower, how you suck his cock, what your snatch tastes like. And he'll assume that you're telling a friend the same kind of things about him: which of his testicles hangs lower, how helpful he is with your orgasms, what the vein on his penis looks like. In case you want to start chatting it up with your people now:

The right testicle, very helpful, and

(← to head to hair →)

During his marriage, Adrian didn't need anyone, didn't want anyone. If he'd had a friend to sex-talk with, it would have gone something like this, "I held my wife's left boob before going to sleep on Friday and I rented a pretty decent porno on Saturday . . . got off twice while she was getting her legs waxed . . . OK, that's all I've got—your turn!"

After so many years of silence, sex-talking with friends after the divorce satisfied some primitive urge in Adrian. He felt like he was a Stone Age hunter huddled around a campfire bragging about his conquests back at the cave. "Here's what we did. Is that weird? Is it not weird enough? Am I missing out on anything?"

Maybe it offends you that Adrian would fuck-and-tell like that. He totally understands how you could feel like your intimacy is being violated when he explains to some third party exactly how your clitoris reacts to this thing or that. But Adrian sees it differently: In exchange for sharing some intimate details, he gets the opportunity to socialize his sexual impulse, sanity-checking that his demands and practices are neither going too far into left field nor becoming too drawn in. He encourages you to do the same and sanity-check your sex life with a friend or two. Be assured that he won't let things get gangbangy or offensive. Though he doesn't have a perfect record in this area, he has generally been discreet.

It might make you feel better to know that, as your relationship stretches from weeks to months, Adrian's sex-talking tapers off in general and he switches from sex-talking to a male friend to sex-talking to a female friend. Not a potential sexual partner, needless to say, but a purely platonic friend. (Adrian has found lesbians and medical professionals to be ideal for this purpose.)

Talking to a woman seems to him not only more respectful but a little healthier. A woman is less likely to encourage a man's most selfish impulses on the order of, "Yeah, she should totally suck your cock in that (and any other imaginable) situation." And might actually contribute some useful information on the order of, "No, she totally wants to suck your cock, she just needs to be approached properly."

Adrian's Nails

Adrian has weak nails. It's not that he hasn't worked to make them stronger. He's tried mixing a gelatin packet in his juice every morning. He's rubbed them with special creams every day. Nothing. Weak nails are just part of the Adrian Colesberry package. Even if he's filed them one evening, he might snag one the next morning and make a sharp edge.

His toenails are the easy part. At least he can keep them out of the way in bed. No such luck for his equally weak fingernails. Years before he would touch his first woman, he developed a full-on paranoia about scratching her soft bits. When the time came, his fear made him a timid finger-fucker and, logically enough, biased him toward eating pussy, since Adrian Colesberry's tongue has no sharp edges on it.

With experience, he learned that a woman's soft bits weren't quite as soft as they'd seemed from the pictures in porn magazines, which made them look like dyed bits of glycerin-moistened tissue paper. Pussy lips didn't bruise to the touch or tear in his hands and by filing his nails to within an inch of their lives, you'll be happy to hear that he got to where he could finger-fuck like a madman with no worries.

Even still, his weak nails may occasionally cause trouble for you as they once caused trouble for the Kind One. One night, she called out from the bathroom, "Did you touch my anus?"

Hearing an earlier-than-anticipated invitation to ass sex, he swaggered, "Yes, I did." Mumbling to himself, "And there's more where that came from!"

She immediately booted him off his cloud, "Oh good, it was bleeding a little bit, I just wanted to make sure that was it." He looked down at his nails and yes, they were a little too long to play around with someone's asshole and a critical one was snaggy. He could have kicked himself. He called out an apology and, while she was still in the bathroom, he trimmed and filed all twenty of his nails to shiny, smooth nubs. By the time she came to bed, he could safely have shoved his big toe up her ass.

Over the next weeks, he set out to reassault his weak-nail problem as he never had before. Be assured that, at this moment, Adrian owns enough equipment to start a nail salon. At his desk, in his car, and in his every backpack and bag, he has a nail clipper, a cuticle trimmer, an orange stick, a file, and a nail buffer. At any moment, in any location, he can tend to a stray cuticle, a snag, or a break. He has even purchased the jewel in the crown of nail salon equipment—a paraffin bath.

If you start having problems with his nails, you might do something imaginative like institute Trim-Your-Fingernails Thursday, where everyone in the whole household sits down, does the paraffin bath, then cuts and files his or her nails. Adrian would appreciate the help.

The Organist

A drian had a gay affair in college.

"This is so typical," the twice-burned reader might be thinking. "Just when I get interested in a man, I find out he's gay."

Now, slow down before you say something you don't mean. That kind of talk is what makes it difficult for men to explore their sexuality. You no doubt have a generous attitude toward same-sex activity but perhaps you also have an unfortunate track record of dating men who are questioning their sexuality and ultimately decide to go the other way. If you're wondering how you've gotten yourself into that pickle again, dog-ear this page and flip back to the front of the book to reread what you wrote in the "Welcome" section about why you wanted to learn how to make love to Adrian Colesberry.

Welcome back. No doubt, your original reasons for wanting to learn how to make love to Adrian Colesberry are just as compelling now that you know about his gay affair back in college as they were when you started.

When Adrian tells you about his gay affair, it's either because he's been with you a while and it's the kind of thing he thinks you should know about or he's intimidated by your greater sexual experience and he's padding his résumé. Thanks to our society's continuing intolerance toward male bisexual behavior, it's great for the latter. A man's ever having taken a cock up his ass trades near the rate of a woman's having a standing Saturday night S/M strap-on orgy with an entire ladies' volleyball squad.

The Great One set a pretty good example of how to react to the news. She didn't appear at all shocked, and to assure him that he hadn't gone too far out on a limb by telling her, she shimmied after him as far as she could—recounting how she'd almost gone lesbian during her radical feminist phase back in college. She'd leaned as far as she could in that direction without following through. She'd hated men's politics and social domination, but she found that she still liked to fuck them.

As much as Adrian would have enjoyed listening to the details of her might-have-been dorm-room lesbian encounters, it was equally nice to hear that even under the formidable pressure of academic feminist dogma, she couldn't give up the cock.

The Great One's response was perfect, but if you wanted to improve on perfection, you could tell Adrian a bit more about your real, near-miss, or imagined experiences with other women.

If you'd like to make something up, but can't quite hack it, maybe the following sentence will get you started.

"I'd been up late studying the night before so I was taking a nap when my roommate came in from an early-morning field hockey practice."

Just seems to write itself from there, but in case you're still stuck, here's the rest of the paragraph: "She had a pretty nasty cut just below her knee and even though we hadn't gotten along all semester, I jumped out of bed without even pulling underwear on to get some iodine and gauze."

Seriously, if you can't take it from there . . .

When Adrian is ready, he'll tell you a version of the story, which goes something, like this: Adrian's first lover, before the Loved One and even before the First One, was a man who had played organ at his church for as long as he could remember. They'd barely said two words to each other when, in his freshman year of college, Adrian ran into him on campus. After talking for a bit, the Organist announced that he had to get to work and asked

Adrian if he wanted to tag along. Having some time on his hands, Adrian did.

The Organist worked at the university museum. Adrian began to visit him there between classes. They talked about art and music and philosophy and Adrian got advice from him about girls, particularly about a girl from church he had a crush on. To appreciate Adrian's level of naiveté at this late age, you should know that he had kissed two girls, each once, in high school and had never had a girlfriend. So to have an older man who had been quite a womanizer earlier in his life offer to be his guide through the world of women seemed quite a plum to Young Adrian.

At some point, the Organist started inviting Adrian to his house and, pretty soon, he was there every weekend. One Saturday, about six months after they'd started their friendship, he kissed Adrian on the lips. Up to that point, Adrian had thought that maybe the Organist could've been gay, but he wasn't 100 percent sure because he'd never come out and said it and besides, he spent so much time giving advice about girls. But when he kissed him . . . Busted! He was totally a fag!

Adrian kissed him back.

It surprised Adrian how great it felt to have someone kissing him. It surprised him that he didn't care about the Organist being a man and that kissing a man wasn't exactly the plan.

The Organist's kissing him opened two great acts in Adrian's young life: his sexual life period, inasmuch as it was expressed with other people, and his quest to figure out whether he was straight or gay. Before he'd kissed a man, Adrian hadn't even thought about it: He'd only ever been attracted to girls in real life; he'd only looked at porn with girls in it. But this kissing a man set off a full-scale investigation of the issue. On the way home that night after their first kiss, he swung by a magazine stand to look at lady porn right alongside guy porn, carefully gauging his reactions to both. He'd never given guy porn a chance, so he had to perform the experiment. He was still only turned on by the girl porn.

Adrian is unlikely to spin into a sexual identity crisis today, regardless of who kisses him. He's older and it's no longer important to him that he's gay or straight or bi or questioning or anything in general. He's less likely to think of himself as a man who likes to fuck women or men or both and more likely to think of himself as a man who likes to fuck the Last One. Some people would say he was bisexual, in the interest of categorizing his behavior. But he never thought of himself that way. He just thought of himself as the guy who liked to fuck the Organist and the Loved One and the Deliberate One and the Talker. That's simpler, isn't it?

Interesting result, but he kept having sex with the Organist. After several months, he ramped up his investigation into the straight-gay thing by losing his virginity to a woman, the First One. After that ended, he got a new girlfriend, the Loved One. But he needed more data, so he started fucking the Deliberate One too and then added the Talker into the mix.

Even to the most ardent, man-loving reader, Adrian might be starting to sound like he's more trouble than he's worth, and the infidelity wasn't the worst of it; he wasn't even a good lover. Adrian was a male version of the Innocent One, which probably explains why he was so patient with her slow acceleration. At least she touched his cock eventually. He barely ever touched the Organist below the shoulders, much less did anything with his penis, and they were together off and on for two years.

It's not that he didn't try to become more active. On the drive over to the Organist's place, he would psych himself up: "This is the day that I'm going to touch his cock, or maybe even give him a blowjob!" While they were having sex, he'd think, "OK . . . Now!" And he'd imagine his elbow bending and his fingers accidentally-on-purpose grazing the Organist's erection. But when he told his arm to move, it wouldn't. Like he was trapped in one of those dreams where you need to run away but are completely paralyzed.

Even in the face of these repeated failures, he kept trying. The way Adrian figured it, once he touched the Organist's penis for the first time, even incidentally, he would magically turn into the cocksucking, handjobbing ass-fucker that he needed to be if he wanted to fully experience the affair that he was having. Didn't happen.

Toward the beginning of his sophomore year, they tried ass-fucking. But Adrian Colesberry wasn't wild about it. Having something in his ass didn't trip him up. That felt good, and in sex, if it feels good, do it. He still enjoys the occasional finger up the ass during a blowjob.

Problem was, Adrian couldn't stay hard while the Organist was fucking him. Throughout the affair, it never became less weird that he was having sex with a guy, but as long as his penis was hard, he took the attitude, "Well, at least someone is having a good time. Who am I to break up a party?" Without his hard-on, it boiled down just to him and a guy's cock up his ass.

When making love to Adrian Colesberry, do make special efforts to keep his penis hard. It does have veto power. Tragically for the Organist, it vetoed ass sex.

Once he started fucking women, it was difficult for Adrian to understand what the Organist saw in him, considering what a lousy lover he was. Even after having one girlfriend, he had developed expectations about what a woman would do for him in bed, but he allowed that poor guy no expectations at all and wondered what he could possibly see in him.

Failure

Adrian broke up with the Organist at the same time as he broke up with all his college girlfriends. In a certain way, ending that relationship bugged him more than the rest because he'd never fully committed to the sexual experience. Homosexual sex is a very popular activity in the world and deserved a better hearing than the one Adrian gave it. The Organist had been a good friend to him in a difficult time. Knowing that he'd be unlikely to pursue another relationship with a man, Adrian really felt like he'd missed the bus by holding back.

His half-baked gayness bugged him mainly on account of his mother's entirely unrealistic vision of him. The good woman spent his entire childhood broadcasting, nonstop, her delusion that he was a genius-in-the-making at everything he put his hand to . . . a fantasy she maintained despite a lot of evidence to the contrary—like his not being good at music or drawing or sports or handwriting.

After hearing enough of her propaganda, he had started believing his own publicity. Imagine then his humiliated confusion when, even after his best efforts, he turned out to be a horrible homosexual.

Adrian viewed his inability to physically love someone of his own sex as a failure of his imagination, a pointless clinging to an outdated and base social morality. He charged himself with being too uncosmopolitan, prudish, and immature to fuck a man without getting all freaked out about his own sexuality.

He argued with himself that just because he loved a man didn't mean that he had to love men for the rest of his life, and just because he was sexually attracted to women, didn't mean that he couldn't love a man. But these glimmers of enlightenment tragically never translated into his mouth around the Organist's cock.

Adrian's Belly Hang-up

If tit-fucking is what you're into, you may be disappointed to hear that it's not Adrian's favorite thing. He'll enjoy it, no doubt, as an occasional bit of nasty fun. But even when tit-fucking for the first time (with the Enthusiast, generous woman that she was) the thrill of novelty was interrupted by a level of discomfort. Everything was going great until he straddled her chest. Before he'd finished one stroke, he looked down to see that his gut was pushed to within inches of the Enthusiast's face. He couldn't get turned on by his cock plowing through her cleavage when he only had eyes for his own belly as it rocked in and out of his visual field.

The ridiculous part is that Adrian didn't even have a big gut at the time. "Why then the upset?" you ask. Well, just as you can't understand Napoleon without knowing that he was short, you can't understand Adrian Colesberry without knowing that Baby Adrian was a little fattie.

His baby fat only survived until puberty. The summer of his thirteenth year, Adrian hit his growth spurt and by the end of that August, he was no longer a little fattie. But fair warning, when tit-fucking, Baby Adrian will charge back onto the scene—as fat and as insecure as ever.

The Enthusiast was busy pressing her boobs together and trying to catch his cock in her mouth at the end of his upstroke. Seriously doubtful that she was thinking about the size of his belly. But so goes the vain insecurity . . . not necessarily of all men, but at least of one man . . . this man, Adrian Colesberry.

Three-Ways

If it's true that more can be learned from failure than from success, then Adrian's experiences with the Enthusiast should be able to teach you everything you need to know about maneuvering Adrian into a three-way. "Hang on!" the sexually adventurous reader might be objecting. "You mean *I* have to maneuver *Adrian* into a three-way? That's not the way it's supposed to work. Does he know that?" No, it's not supposed to work that way. And yes, he does know it.

In an ideal world, after Adrian meets a barista or waitress or your friend or cousin (not your first cousin or you'd have to get permission from the pope), *he's* the one who's supposed to start pestering *you*, "Hey, this/your barista/waitress/friend/cousin is pretty hot. Wouldn't it be super-sexy if the three of us all fucked one another at the same time?" Then you throw up some token resistance to retain your reputation for modesty and right thinking until, finally, you submit to his artless pleading and help him arrange it so that you two can fuck this other lady, whoever she is.

Unhappily, this is not an ideal world. And as much as Adrian might want to be the guy who can convince himself that the best thing for you personally and for your future life together with him would be to bring another lady into orbit around his cock, he's somehow not motivated to pursue this as a sexual goal. But just because Adrian won't be trying to make you jump into bed with every woman who gives him an erection, that doesn't mean he won't fuck your friend if you want him to. Especially since you can succeed where the Enthusiast failed by learning from her mistakes.

Mistake No. 1: Tell Adrian nothing about your plans

One weekend, the Enthusiast asked Adrian if he'd help her throw a birthday party for a friend. He agreed of course and, come Saturday night, there they sat around the woman's coffee table. As the friend opened her candles and cards, the Enthusiast turned the conversation to her friend's stunning good looks, asking Adrian several times what he thought of her beauty, her body, and begging him to explain "why, oh why," a man had not snatched her up yet. Adrian complimented the friend's various assets and apologized for the incomprehensible disinterest of his sex, but still he did not catch on to the plot that the Enthusiast was hatching, where the girls would end the evening tag-teaming his cock.

From this obtuseness, do not conclude that Adrian does not admire and aspire toward the three-way. It is, after all, one of the holy trinity of non-fetishy male perversions, the other two being on-tap blowjobs and ass sex.

Give him some advance warning and Adrian will work to help you reach the ultimate goal you have in mind. Give him no warning, and things will go wrong, as they did with the Enthusiast.

Mistake No. 2: Pick a friend who doesn't really like you

If you want Adrian to fuck another lady with you, make sure the lady at least acts like she likes you. That way he'll be able to guess what you're up to. And by all means, don't carry on some low-grade squabble the whole evening. Adrian's three-way fantasy doesn't involve two she-wolves snarling over him.

There was a tension between the two so-called friends pretty much from the beginning, and the friend got grumpier as she got drunker. The Enthusiast more or less spent the evening apologizing for this, that, and the other. In these circumstances, Adrian wasn't entertaining any hopes that the girls would end up making out with each other. On top of this, Adrian does have a sense of loyalty: If the friend wanted access to his cock, she shouldn't have been snarky toward the woman who was regularly sucking on it.

Mistake No. 3: Get Adrian pissing drunk

Decide which one you want to do: get Adrian super drunk or have him fuck you and your friend. He can't do both. To be fair, it wasn't the Enthusiast's fault if she thought Adrian would hold up under the effects of alcohol. Aside from the mornings, they had never fucked sober. The difference-maker in this situation was that between *Adrian domesticus* and *Adrian economicus*.

Sitting on her couch all those evenings, he hadn't felt obliged to finish each pitcher of martinis that she made, as bottles of vodka are pretty cheap. But on that evening's bar crawl through the downtown of the suburban community where the friend lived, the drinks were anything but cheap, and when the Enthusiast insisted on buying round after round, he felt like he would have been burning money if he didn't finish the cocktails, so he did—down to the dregs. Passing out was the only thing he was fit to do once they finally ended up back at the friend's apartment after last call.

Don't be worried that Adrian has a drinking problem. He'd much rather fuck than drink, so especially on a date, he carefully controls his alcohol consumption. He'll down two or three cocktails at the beginning of the evening then switch to water for the duration. That way, when it's time for you two to head home, he's sober for the drive and for the fucking. You will in no way have to monitor Adrian's drinking when you go out, just don't tirelessly ply him with drinks, because he will drink them and then will be too drunk to fuck you, much less your friend.

Mistake No. 4: Once the sex starts, don't participate in any way

What Adrian looks forward to in a three-way is some light (or full-on but no pressure) lesbotic activity between the girls that he can insert himself into. Under no circumstances should you set up some situation where one of you is just watching, like the Enthusiast did. (Although if you wanted to fuck your girlfriend while Adrian watched, that would be terrific.)

When they got back to the girl's house, Adrian somehow ended up lying on his back on the kitchen floor with someone straddling his crotch. He thought that someone was the Enthusiast, naturally enough, but when his eyes focused, it turned out to be the friend. He rolled his head around to find the Enthusiast, and when he did she was leaning in the entrance to the kitchen, watching the two of them like they were a top she'd set spinning and she was disinterestedly curious as to where they'd end up.

That's when he finally caught on for sure that the woman's real gift that evening wasn't the soaps or the candles or the free all-you-can-drink alcohol. Her real gift was Adrian Colesberry. She'd wanted to go out on her birthday and get drunk and get fucked and the Enthusiast had brought him in to do the fucking.

Only by this time he was way too drunk so, after an awkward minute, the friend rolled off him and stormed out of the room. Even sober he would have been disinclined to fuck this grumpy lady.

To summarize, the four steps to your fantasy three-way with Adrian Colesberry are as follows: 1. Get him involved in the planning; 2. Make sure that you and your girlfriend are flirty or at least nice to each other during the execution phase; 3. Don't let him get too drunk, although a little drunk is probably necessary; 4. No spectators, with the possible exception of Adrian Colesberry.

You are totally capable of pulling this off.

Losing His Virginity

Adrian's unwelcomed virginity survived high school and kept him company partway through college. Then in the middle of his sophomore year, he moved out of his parents' place and into the back room of a house near the university. New Year's Eve day, he lugged over his last carload of stuff. New Year's Eve, he and his new roommates threw a party. And on New Year's Day, at two o'clock in the morning, he gave away his virginity, following an age-old tradition for incompetent boys, to a fat slut.

It was after midnight and Adrian was hanging out on the porch when a girl he hadn't noticed during the New Year's party came up to him. She had an average figure from the navel up. It was her hips! They jutted out at nearly right angles from her torso. You could have securely rested a beer mug on the shelf they created.

Without even introducing herself, the girl on the porch said, "Would you like to come home and see my pussy?"

He learned later that she'd put the same question to every guy at the party. Having struck out with them, she decided to take one last swing with Adrian on her way out the door. As it happened, one of the things Adrian wanted to do that year was lose his virginity so, needless to say, he agreed to follow her home.

When they walked into her place, the First One got this devilish look on her face and introduced him to her cat. Adrian felt a bit stung. "Come home and see my pussy" was a terrible pun and something of an old joke. Still, he didn't lose his spirit one bit.

Having never had girlfriends in high school, he didn't know anything to do but just kiss her. Even after she took her top off, he didn't try to get to second base—her boobs naked right there in front of him. They made out like that for over an hour. He would have kept at it, but finally the First One came up for air and asked, "Are you a virgin?"

Reflexively, he denied it, "Me?! No way!" But from the look in her eyes, he could tell that she didn't believe him. He'd played enough penny-ante poker to know that he couldn't get away with even the smallest bluff, so, not wanting to embarrass himself any more than he already had, he just fessed up. "OK. Yes, I'm a virgin. Can we still have sex?"

She thought for a while, then explained. "No, I've deflowered guys before. It always gets messy. I just don't feel like it right now."

Understood. It wasn't her job to provide that service for him and he wasn't going to beg. So he just asked, "Can we keep making out?" And that's the line that got his cherry popped.

After five more minutes of foreplay, the First One lay on her back, hiked her knees up to her armpits, and pulled him on top of her—all in one fluid motion. Once in position, she reached down, found his erection, which was poking her in the stomach at the time, and efficiently fit his cock inside her. She had definitely done this before. Adrian Colesberry got a smug feeling, the kind you get when you've picked a competent auto mechanic: "Everything's going to work out just fine."

INDEX

Note: Page numbers in *italics* denote charts, graphs, and illustrations. The abbreviation "AC" refers to Adrian Colesberry.